Health Science and Alternative Health Care

Health Science and Alternative Health Care

Shailendra Sengar

ANMOL PUBLICATIONS PVT. LTD.
NEW DELHI-110 002 (INDIA)

ANMOL PUBLICATIONS PVT. LTD.
H.O.: 4374/4B, Ansari Road, Darya Ganj,
New Delhi-110 002 (India)
Ph.: 23278000, 23261597
B.O.: No. 1015, Ist Main Road, BSK IIIrd Stage
IIIrd Phase, IIIrd Block
Bangalore - 560 085 (India)
Visit us at: www.anmolpublications.com

Health Science and Alternative Health Care

First Published, 2008

ISBN 978-81-261-3433-5

PRINTED IN INDIA

Printed at Mehra Offset Press, Delhi.

Contents

Preface

This Encyclopaedic Series of Career and Vocational Guidance Covers careers, describing jobs, places of employment, working conditions, qualifications, education and training. This has been developed to aid career and counsellors and job placement coordinators in planning activities for students and potential students about career vocational education programs. It contains a career and vocational guidance model which clarifies what career and vocational guidance services mean and what planners should include in their activities. The model shows an interrelatedness among major thrusts with career development being a central theme of vocational guidance. All of the thrusts depicted in the model represent essential services that should be available to students in career and vocational education programs. The encyclopaedia deals with various sections which correspond to the major thrusts identified in the model: (1) career development; (2) recruitment; (3) guidance and counselling; (4) placement; (5) follow-up and follow-through; and (6) consultation. Each section contains an outline of the perceived needs of the topic, an overview of the topic relative to career and vocational guidance, and some suggested activities and strategies that may be useful in meeting student needs.

It also contains current information about occupations, employment trends, and job searching. Materials on career decision-making, internships, and salaries are also located in each volume. This Series of Encyclopaedia helps students assess their potential for various careers.

Shailendra Sengar

1

Career in Health Science

Medicine and Dentistry

Your girlfriend asked you what makes you tick. And there, you launched into an elaborate explanation which went like this: the heart, of course, which is a muscular pump, beats about 72 times a minute through a continuous and automatic process of muscular contraction and relaxation. Hey, why don't you give medicine a shot? Maybe that is where your heart is!

On a less frivolous note, medicine is about healing. It is a noble profession, for which one needs to study physics, chemistry and biology (PCB) at the 10+2 level and take competitive entrance exams to gain admission to institutes offering MBBS degrees.

Broadly speaking, an aspirant in the field of medicine can take up:

- Allopathic medicine
- Homeopathy
- Dentistry
- Veterinary science
- Other alternative systems of medicine such as Ayurveda.

In medical practice, general medicine is an umbrella term for a large number of specialized fields of study. For example a general practitioner if interested in the peculiarities of human behaviour can choose to specialize in psychiatry.

We have information on:

- Medicine and Dentistry

- Pharmacy
- Physiotherapy
- Orthotic technology
- Nursing

Each career carries an extensive list of institutes with addresses in the where to study section. Hope this helps your career take shape.

Psychologists

Significant Points: About 4 out of 10 psychologists are self-employed, compared with less than 1 out of 10 among all professional workers.

Most specialists, including clinical and counselling psychologists, need a doctoral degree; school psychologists need an educational specialist degree and industrial-organizational psychologists need a master's degree.

Competition for admission to graduate psychology programmes is keen.

Overall employment of psychologists is expected to grow faster than the average for all occupations through 2014.

Nature of the Work: Psychologists study the human mind and human behaviour. Research psychologists investigate the physical, cognitive, emotional, or social aspects of human behaviour. Psychologists in health service provider fields provide mental health care in hospitals, clinics, schools, or private settings. Psychologists employed in applied settings, such as business, industry, government, or non-profits, provide training, conduct research, design systems and act as advocates for psychology.

Like other social scientists, psychologists formulate hypotheses and collect data to test their validity. Research methods vary with the topic under study. Psychologists sometimes gather information through controlled laboratory experiments or by administering personality, performance, aptitude, or intelligence tests. Other methods include observation, interviews, questionnaires, clinical studies and surveys.

Psychologists apply their knowledge to a wide range of endeavours, including health and human services, management, education, law and sports. In addition to working in a variety of settings, psychologists usually specialize in one of a number of different areas.

Clinical psychologists—who constitute the largest speciality—work most often in counselling centres, independent or group practices, hospitals, or clinics. They help mentally and emotionally disturbed clients adjust to life and may assist medical and surgical patients in dealing with illnesses or injuries. Some clinical psychologists work in physical rehabilitation settings, treating patients with spinal cord injuries, chronic pain or illness, stroke, arthritis and neurological conditions. Others help people deal with times of personal crisis, such as divorce or the death of a loved one.

Clinical psychologists often interview patients and give diagnostic tests. They may provide individual, family, or group psychotherapy and may design and implement behaviour modification programmes.

Some clinical psychologists collaborate with physicians and other specialists to develop and implement treatment and intervention programmes that patients can understand and comply with. Other clinical psychologists work in universities and medical schools, where they train graduate students in the delivery of mental health and behavioural medicine services. Some administer community mental health programmes.

Areas of specialization within clinical psychology include health psychology, neuropsychology and geropsychology. *Health psychologists* promote good health through health maintenance counselling programmes designed to help people achieve goals, such as stopping smoking or losing weight. *Neuropsychologists* study the relation between the brain and behaviour.

They often work in stroke and head injury programmes. *Geropsychologists* deal with the special problems faced by the elderly. The emergence and growth of these specialities reflects the increasing participation of psychologists in providing direct services to special patient populations.

Often, clinical psychologists will consult with other medical personnel regarding the best treatment for patients, especially treatment that includes medication. Clinical psychologists generally are not permitted to prescribe medication to treat patients; only psychiatrists and other medical doctors may prescribe certain medications. However, two States—Louisiana and New Mexico—currently allow clinical psychologists to prescribe medication with some limitations and similar proposals have been made in other States.

Counselling psychologists use various techniques, including interviewing and testing, to advise people on how to deal with problems of everyday living. They work in settings such as university counselling centres, hospitals and individual or group practices. (See also the statements on counsellors and social workers elsewhere in the *Handbook*.)

School psychologists work with students in elementary and secondary schools. They collaborate with teachers, parents and school personnel to create safe, healthy and supportive learning environments for all students; address students' learning and behaviour problems; improve classroom management strategies or parenting skills; counter substance abuse; assess students with learning disabilities and gifted and talented students to help determine the best way to educate them; and improve teaching, learning and socialization strategies.

They also may evaluate the effectiveness of academic programmes, prevention programmes, behaviour management procedures and other services provided in the school setting. *Industrial-organizational psychologists* apply psychological principles and research methods to the workplace in the interest of improving productivity and the quality of worklife. They also are involved in research on management and marketing problems. They screen, train and counsel applicants for jobs, as well as perform organizational development and analysis. An industrial psychologist might work with management to reorganize the work setting in order to improve productivity or quality of life in the workplace. Industrial psychologists frequently act as consultants, brought in by management to solve a particular problem.

Developmental psychologists study the physiological, cognitive and social development that takes place throughout life. Some specialize in behaviour during infancy, childhood and adolescence, or changes that occur during maturity or old age. Developmental psychologists also may study developmental disabilities and their effects. Increasingly, research is developing ways to help elderly people remain independent as long as possible.

Social psychologists examine people's interactions with others and with the social environment. They work in organizational consultation, marketing research, systems design, or other applied psychology fields. Prominent areas of study include group behaviour, leadership, attitudes and perception.

Experimental or *research psychologists* work in university and private research centres and in business, non-profit and governmental organizations. They study the behaviour of both human beings and animals, such as rats, monkeys and pigeons. Prominent areas of study in experimental research include motivation, thought, attention, learning and memory, sensory and perceptual processes, effects of substance abuse and genetic and neurological factors affecting behaviour.

Working Conditions: A psychologist's sub-field and place of employment determine his or her working conditions. Clinical, school and counselling psychologists in private practice have their own offices and set their own hours. However, they often offer evening and weekend hours to accommodate their clients. Those employed in hospitals, nursing homes and other health care facilities may work shifts that include evenings and weekends, while those who work in schools and clinics generally work regular hours.

Psychologists employed as faculty by colleges and universities divide their time between teaching and research and also may have administrative responsibilities; many have part-time consulting practices. Most psychologists in government and industry have structured schedules.

Increasingly, many psychologists are working as part of a team, consulting with other psychologists and professionals.

Many experience pressures because of deadlines, tight schedules and overtime. Their routine may be interrupted frequently. Travel may be required in order to attend conferences or conduct research.

Training, Other Qualifications and Advancement: A doctoral degree usually is required for employment as an independent licensed clinical or counselling psychologist. Psychologists with a Ph.D. qualify for a wide range of teaching, research, clinical and counselling positions in universities, health care services, elementary and secondary schools, private industry and government. Psychologists with a Doctor of Psychology (Psy.D.) degree usually work in clinical positions or in private practices, but they also sometime teach, conduct research, or carry out administrative responsibilities.

A doctoral degree generally requires 5 to 7 years of graduate study. The Ph.D. degree culminates in a dissertation based on original research. Courses in quantitative research methods, which include the use of computer-based analysis, are an integral part of graduate study and are necessary to complete the dissertation. The Psy.D. may be based on practical work and examinations rather than a dissertation. In clinical or counselling psychology, the requirements for the doctoral degree include at least a 1-year internship.

A specialist degree is required in most States for an individual to work as a school psychologist, although a few States still credential school psychologists with master's degrees. A specialist (Ed.S.) degree in school psychology requires a minimum of 3 years of full-time graduate study (at least 60 graduate semester hours) and a 1-year internship. Because their professional practice addresses educational and mental health components of students' development, school psychologists' training includes coursework in both education and psychology.

Persons with a master's degree in psychology may work as industrial-organizational psychologists. They also may work as psychological assistants under the supervision of doctoral-level psychologists and may conduct research or psychological evaluations. A master's degree in psychology requires at least two years of full-time graduate study. Requirements usually include practical experience in an applied setting and a master's thesis based on an original research project.

Competition for admission to graduate psychology programmes is keen. Some universities require applicants to have an undergraduate major in psychology. Others prefer only coursework in basic psychology with courses in the biological, physical and social sciences and in statistics and mathematics.

A bachelor's degree in psychology qualifies a person to assist psychologists and other professionals in community mental health centres, vocational rehabilitation offices and correctional programmes. Bachelor's degree holders may work as research or administrative assistants for psychologists. Some work as technicians in related fields, such as marketing research. Many find employment in other areas, such as sales or business management.

In the Federal Government, candidates having at least 24 semester hours in psychology and one course in statistics qualify for entry-level positions. However, competition for these jobs is keen because this is one of the few areas in which one can work as a psychologist without an advanced degree.

The American Psychological Association (APA) presently accredits doctoral training programmes in clinical, counselling and school psychology, as well as accrediting institutions that provide internships for doctoral students in school, clinical and counselling psychology. The National Association of School Psychologists, with the assistance of the National Council for Accreditation of Teacher Education, also is involved in the accreditation of advanced degree programmes in school psychology.

Psychologists in independent practice or those who offer any type of patient care—including clinical, counselling and school psychologists—must meet certification or licensing requirements in all States and the Districts of Columbia. Licensing laws vary by State and by type of position and require licensed or certified psychologists to limit their practice to areas in which they have developed professional competence through training and experience. Clinical and counselling psychologists usually require a doctorate in psychology, the completion of an approved internship and 1 to 2 years of professional experience.

In addition, all States require that applicants pass an examination. Most State licensing boards administer a standardized test and many supplement that with additional oral or essay questions. Some States require continuing education for renewal of the license.

The National Association of School Psychologists (NASP) awards the Nationally Certified School Psychologist (NCSP) designation, which recognizes professional competency in school psychology at a national, rather than State, level. Currently, 26 States recognize the NCSP and allow those with the certification to transfer credentials from one State to another without taking a new certification exam. In States that recognize the NCSP, the requirements for certification or licensure and those for the NCSP often are the same or similar. Requirements for the NCSP include the completion of 60 graduate semester hours in school psychology; a 1,200-hour internship, 600 hours of which must be completed in a school setting; and a passing score on the National School Psychology Examination.

The American Board of Professional Psychology (ABPP) recognizes professional achievement by awarding speciality certification, primarily in clinical psychology, clinical neuropsychology and counselling, forensic, industrial-organizational and school psychology. Candidates for ABPP certification need a doctorate in psychology, post-doctoral training in their speciality, five years of experience, professional endorsements and a passing grade on an examination.

Aspiring psychologists who are interested in direct patient care must be emotionally stable, mature and able to deal effectively with people. Sensitivity, compassion, good communication skills and the ability to lead and inspire others are particularly important qualities for persons wishing to do clinical work and counselling. Research psychologists should be able to do detailed work both independently and as part of a team. Patience and perseverance are vital qualities, because achieving results in the psychological treatment of patients or in research may take a long time.

Employment: Psychologists held about 179,000 jobs in 2004. Educational institutions employed about 1 out of 4 psychologists in positions other than teaching, such as counselling, testing, research and administration. Almost 2 out of 10 were employed in health care, primarily in offices of mental health practitioners, physicians' offices, outpatient mental health and substance abuse centres and private hospitals. Government agencies at the State and local levels employed psychologists in public hospitals, clinics, correctional facilities and other settings.

After several years of experience, some psychologists—usually those with doctoral degrees—enter private practice or set up private research or consulting firms. About 4 out of 10 psychologists were self-employed in 2004, compared with less than 1 out of 10 among all professional workers.

In addition to the previously mentioned jobs, many psychologists held faculty positions at colleges and universities and as high school psychology teachers. (See the statements on teachers—post-secondary and teachers—preschool, kindergarten, elementary, middle and secondary elsewhere in the *Handbook*.)

Job Outlook: Employment of psychologists is expected to grow faster than average for all occupations through 2014, because of increased demand for psychological services in schools, hospitals, social service agencies, mental health centres, substance abuse treatment clinics, consulting firms and private companies.

Among the specialities in this field, school psychologists—especially those with a specialist degree or higher—may enjoy the best job opportunities. Growing awareness of how students' mental health and behavioural problems, such as bullying, affect learning is increasing demand for school psychologists to offer student counselling and mental health services. Clinical and counselling psychologists will be needed to help people deal with depression and other mental disorders, marriage and family problems, job stress and addiction. The rise in health care costs associated with unhealthy lifestyles, such as smoking, alcoholism and obesity, has made prevention and treatment more critical. An increase in the number of employee assistance programmes, which help workers deal with personal problems, also should spur job growth in clinical and counselling specialities. Industrial-organizational psychologists will be in demand to help to boost worker productivity and retention rates in a wide range of businesses. Industrial-organizational psychologists will help companies deal with issues such as workplace diversity and anti-discrimination policies. Companies also will use psychologists' expertise in survey design, analysis and research to develop tools for marketing evaluation and statistical analysis.

Demand should be particularly strong for persons holding doctorates from leading universities in applied specialities—such as counselling, health and school psychology. Psychologists with extensive training in quantitative research methods and computer science may have a competitive edge over applicants without background.

Master's degree holders in fields other than industrial-organizational psychology will face keen competition for jobs, because of the limited number of positions that require only a master's degree. Master's degree holders may find jobs as psychological assistants or counsellors, providing mental health services under the direct supervision of a licensed psychologist. Still others may find jobs involving research and data collection and analysis in universities, government, or private companies.

Opportunities directly related to psychology will be limited for bachelor's degree holders. Some may find jobs as assistants in rehabilitation centres or in other jobs involving data collection and analysis. Those who meet State certification requirements may become high school psychology teachers.

Earnings: Median annual earnings of wage and salary clinical, counselling and school psychologists in May 2004 were \$54,950. The middle 50 percent earned between \$41,850 and \$71,880. The lowest 10 percent earned less than \$32,280 and the highest 10 percent earned more than \$92,250. Median annual earnings in the industries employing the largest numbers of clinical, counselling and school psychologists in May 2004 were:

Offices of other health practitioners	$64,460
Elementary and secondary schools	58,360
Outpatient care centres	46,850
Individual and family services	42,640

Median annual earnings of wage and salary industrial-organizational psychologists in May 2004 were $71,400. The middle 50 percent earned between $56,880 and $93,210. The lowest 10 percent earned less than $45,620 and the highest 10 percent earned more than $125,560.

Medical Technology

Medical technologists are behind-the-scenes workers in the medical profession. Using sophisticated diagnostic and therapeutic equipment, they are trained to make and report investigations providing tremendous assistance to the medical practitioners in their work with patients. With the development of a variety of equipment, the need for skilled technicians and other trained paramedical personnel has increased in the recent years.

Orthotic Technology

Prosthetic and Orthotic Engineering is a medico-engineering profession, which deals with physically disabled, crippled and orthopaedically handicapped persons. Patients who have lost a limb in an accident or since birth, or are crippled due to diseases like polio, encephalitis etc. are rehabilitated by providing artificial replacements such as calipers, splints or artificial limbs. Today, this branch is well developed and uses the latest technology and materials for preparing artificial limbs.

Orthotists work with patients with limb or spine related disabilities. The study programme of Orthotics and Prosthetics includes anatomy, orthopaedics, amputational surgery and immediate post surgical prothesis. The engineering aspects of the course include subjects such as applied mechanics and kinethesiology.

Pharmacy

Pharmacists study the chemistry of drugs, their origin, procedures for drug development, their preparation, dispensing, their effects and eventual use for prevention and treatment of disease. The complexity of drug therapy and the dangers of drug abuse has brought into focus the need of pharmacists' special skills to maintain a rational approach in the realm of drug treatments.

Pharmacists work in research, processing and manufacture of drugs. Biotechnological research has added a dynamic potential to the work of pharmacists. The investment in research and development is envisaged to expand the sphere of business activity, both in the country and abroad. Multinational joint venture partnerships have given a thrust to this growth, which has targeted business of almost 40,000 crores, approximately 3.8% of the market share by the turn of the century.

Pharmacists

Significant Points: Very good employment opportunities are expected for pharmacists.

Earnings are high, but some pharmacists work long hours, nights, weekends and holidays.

Pharmacists are becoming more involved in making decisions regarding drug therapy and in counselling patients.

A license is required; the prospective pharmacist must graduate from an accredited college of pharmacy and pass a State examination.

Nature of the Work: Pharmacists distribute drugs prescribed by physicians and other health practitioners and provide information to patients about medications and their use. They advise physicians and other health practitioners on the selection, dosages, interactions and side effects of medications. Pharmacists also monitor the health and progress of patients in response to drug therapy to ensure the safe and effective use of medication. Pharmacists must understand the use, clinical effects and composition of drugs, including their chemical, biological and physical properties. Compounding—

the actual mixing of ingredients to form powders, tablets, capsules, ointments and solutions—is a small part of a pharmacist's practice, because most medicines are produced by pharmaceutical companies in a standard dosage and drug delivery form. Most pharmacists work in a community setting, such as a retail drugstore, or in a health care facility, such as a hospital, nursing home, mental health institution, or neighborhood health clinic.

Pharmacists in community and retail pharmacies counsel patients and answer questions about prescription drugs, including questions regarding possible side effects or interactions among various drugs. They provide information about over-the-counter drugs and make recommendations after talking with the patient.

They also may give advice about the patient's diet, exercise, or stress management or about durable medical equipment and home health care supplies. In addition, they also may complete third-party insurance forms and other paperwork. Those who own or manage community pharmacies may sell non-health-related merchandise, hire and supervise personnel and oversee the general operation of the pharmacy.

Some community pharmacists provide specialized services to help patients manage conditions such as diabetes, asthma, smoking cessation, or high blood pressure. Some community pharmacists also are trained to administer vaccinations.

Pharmacists in health care facilities dispense medications and advise the medical staff on the selection and effects of drugs. They may make sterile solutions to be administered intravenously. They also assess, plan and monitor drug programmes or regimens. Pharmacists counsel hospitalized patients on the use of drugs and on their use at home when the patients are discharged. Pharmacists also may evaluate drug-use patterns and outcomes for patients in hospitals or managed care organizations.

Pharmacists who work in home health care monitor drug therapy and prepare infusions—solutions that are injected into patients—and other medications for use in the home.

Some pharmacists specialize in specific drug therapy areas, such as intravenous nutrition support, oncology (cancer), nuclear pharmacy (used for chemotherapy), geriatric pharmacy and psychopharmacotherapy (the treatment of mental disorders by means of drugs).

Most pharmacists keep confidential computerized records of patients' drug therapies to prevent harmful drug interactions. Pharmacists are responsible for the accuracy of every prescription that is filled, but they often rely upon pharmacy technicians and pharmacy aides to assist them in the dispensing process. Thus, the pharmacist may delegate prescription-filling and administrative tasks and supervise their completion. Pharmacists also frequently oversee pharmacy students serving as interns in preparation for graduation and licensure.

Increasingly, pharmacists are pursuing nontraditional pharmacy work. Some are involved in research for pharmaceutical manufacturers, developing new drugs and therapies and testing their effects on people. Others work in marketing or sales, providing expertise to clients on a drug's use, effectiveness and possible side effects.

Some pharmacists work for health insurance companies, developing pharmacy benefit packages and carrying out cost-benefit analyses on certain drugs. Other pharmacists work for the government, public health care services, the armed services and pharmacy associations. Finally, some pharmacists are employed full time or part time as college faculty, teaching classes and performing research in a wide range of areas.

Working Conditions: Pharmacists work in clean, well-lighted and well-ventilated areas. Many pharmacists spend most of their workday on their feet. When working with sterile or dangerous pharmaceutical products, pharmacists wear gloves and masks and work with other special protective equipment. Many community and hospital pharmacies are open for extended hours or around the clock, so pharmacists may work nights, weekends and holidays. Consultant pharmacists may travel to nursing homes or other facilities to monitor patients' drug therapy.

About 21 percent of pharmacists worked part time in 2004. Most full-time salaried pharmacists worked approximately 40 hours a week. Some, including many self-employed pharmacists, worked more than 50 hours a week.

Training, Other Qualifications and Advancement: A license to practice pharmacy is required in all States, the District of Columbia and all U.S. territories. To obtain a license, the prospective pharmacist must graduate from a college of pharmacy that is accredited by the Accreditation Council for Pharmacy Education (ACPE) and pass an examination. All States require the North American Pharmacist Licensure Exam (NAPLEX), which tests pharmacy skills and knowledge and 43 states and the District of Columbia require the Multistate Pharmacy Jurisprudence Exam (MPJE), which tests pharmacy law.

Both exams are administered by the National Association of Boards of Pharmacy. Pharmacists in the eight states that do not require the MJPE must pass a state-specific exam that is similar to the MJPE. In addition to the NAPLEX and MPJE, some States require additional exams unique to their State. All States except California currently grant a license without extensive re-examination to qualified pharmacists who already are licensed by another State.

In Florida, re-examination is not required if a pharmacist has passed the NAPLEX and MPJE within 12 years of his or her application for a license transfer. Many pharmacists are licensed to practice in more than one State. Most States require continuing education for license renewal. Persons interested in a career as a pharmacist should check with individual State boards of pharmacy for details on examination requirements, license renewal requirements and license transfer procedures.

In 2004, 89 colleges of pharmacy were accredited to confer degrees by the Accreditation Council for Pharmacy Education. Pharmacy programmes grant the degree of Doctor of Pharmacy (Pharm.D.), which requires at least 6 years of post-secondary study and the passing of a State board of pharmacy's licensure examination. Courses offered at colleges of pharmacy are designed to teach students about all aspects of drug therapy.

In addition, schools teach students how to communicate with patients and other health care providers about drug information and patient care. Students also learn professional ethics, how to develop and manage medication distribution systems and concepts of public health. In addition to receiving classroom instruction, students in Pharm.D. programmes spend about one-forth of their time learning in a variety of pharmacy practice settings under the supervision of licensed pharmacists. The Pharm.D. degree has replaced the Bachelor of Pharmacy (B.Pharm.) degree, which is no longer being awarded.

The Pharm.D. is a 4-year programme that requires at least 2 years of college study prior to admittance, although most applicants have completed 3 years. Entry requirements usually include courses in mathematics and natural sciences, such as chemistry, biology and physics, as well as courses in the humanities and social sciences. Approximately two-thirds of all colleges require applicants to take the Pharmacy College Admissions Test (PCAT).

In 2003, the American Association of Colleges of Pharmacy (AACP) launched the Pharmacy College Application Service, known as PharmCAS, for students who are interested in applying to schools and colleges of pharmacy. This centralized service allows applicants to use a single Web-based application and one set of transcripts to apply to multiple schools of pharmacy. A total of 43 schools participated in 2003.

In the 2003–04 academic year, 67 colleges of pharmacy awarded the master-of-science degree or the Ph.D. degree. Both degrees are awarded after the completion of a Pharm.D. degree and are designed for those who want more laboratory and research experience. Many master's and Ph.D. degree holders do research for a drug company or teach at a university. Other options for pharmacy graduates who are interested in further training include 1-year or 2-year residency programmes or fellowships. Pharmacy residencies are postgraduate training programmes in pharmacy practice and usually require the completion of a research study. There currently are more than 700 residency training programmes nationwide. Pharmacy fellowships are highly individualized programmes that are designed to prepare participants to work in a specialized area of pharmacy, such clinical practice or research laboratories. Some pharmacists who run their own pharmacy obtain a master's degree in business administration (MBA). Others may obtain a degree in public administration or public health.

Areas of graduate study include pharmaceutics and pharmaceutical chemistry (physical and chemical properties of drugs and dosage forms), pharmacology (effects of drugs on the body), toxicology and pharmacy administration.

Prospective pharmacists should have scientific aptitude, good communication skills and a desire to help others. They also must be conscientious and pay close attention to detail, because the decisions they make affect human lives.

In community pharmacies, pharmacists usually begin at the staff level. In independent pharmacies, after they gain experience and secure the necessary capital, some become owners or part owners of pharmacies. Pharmacists in chain drugstores may be promoted to pharmacy supervisor or manager at the store level, then to manager at the district or regional level and later to an executive position within the chain's headquarters.

Hospital pharmacists may advance to supervisory or administrative positions. Pharmacists in the pharmaceutical industry may advance in marketing, sales, research, quality control, production, packaging, or other areas.

Employment: Pharmacists held about 230,000 jobs in 2004. About 61 percent work in community pharmacies that are either independently owned or part of a drugstore chain, grocery store, department store, or mass merchandiser. Most community pharmacists are salaried employees, but some are self-employed owners. About 24 percent of salaried pharmacists work in hospitals. Others work in clinics, mail-order pharmacies, pharmaceutical wholesalers, home health care agencies, or the Federal Government.

Job Outlook: Very good employment opportunities are expected for pharmacists over the 2004–14 period because the number of job openings created by employment growth and the need to replace pharmacists who leave the occupation or retire are expected to exceed the number of degrees granted in pharmacy. Enrollments in pharmacy programmes are rising as more students are attracted by high salaries and good job prospects. Despite this increase in enrollments, job openings should still be more numerous than those seeking employment.

Employment of pharmacists is expected to grow faster than the average for all occupations through the year 2014, because of the increasing demand for pharmaceuticals, particularly from the growing elderly population. The increasing numbers of middle-aged and elderly people—who use more prescription drugs than younger people—will continue to spur demand for pharmacists in all employment settings.

Other factors likely to increase the demand for pharmacists include scientific advances that will make more drug products available, new developments in genome research and medication distribution systems, increasingly sophisticated consumers seeking more information about drugs and coverage of prescription drugs by a greater number of health insurance plans and Medicare.

Community pharmacies are taking steps to manage an increasing volume of prescriptions. Automation of drug dispensing and greater employment of pharmacy technicians and pharmacy aides will help these establishments to dispense more prescriptions.

With its emphasis on cost control, managed care encourages the use of lower cost prescription drug distributors, such as mail-order firms and online pharmacies, for purchases of certain medications. Prescriptions ordered through the mail and via the internet are filled in a central location and shipped to the patient at a lower cost. Mail-order and online pharmacies typically use automated technology to dispense medication and employ fewer pharmacists. If the utilization of mail-order pharmacies increases rapidly, job growth among pharmacists could be limited.

Employment of pharmacists will not grow as fast in hospitals as in other industries, because hospitals are reducing inpatient stays, downsizing and consolidating departments. The number of outpatient surgeries is increasing, so more patients are being discharged and purchasing their medications through retail, supermarket, or mail-order pharmacies, rather than through hospitals. An aging population means that more pharmacy services will be required in nursing homes, assisted-living facilities and home care settings. The most rapid job growth among pharmacists is expected in these 3 settings.

New opportunities are emerging for pharmacists in managed care organizations where they analyze trends and patterns in medication use and in pharmacoeconomics—the cost and benefit analysis of different drug therapies. Opportunities also are emerging for pharmacists trained in research and disease management—the development of new methods for curing and controlling diseases. Pharmacists also are finding jobs in research and development and in sales and marketing for pharmaceutical manufacturing firms.

New breakthroughs in biotechnology will increase the potential for drugs to treat diseases and expand the opportunities for pharmacists to conduct research and sell medications. In addition, pharmacists are finding employment opportunities in pharmacy informatics, which uses information technology to improve patient care.

Job opportunities for pharmacists in patient care will arise as cost-conscious insurers and health systems continue to emphasize the role of pharmacists in primary and preventive health care. Health insurance companies realize that the expense of using medication to treat diseases and various health conditions often is considerably less than the costs for patients whose conditions go untreated. Pharmacists also can reduce the expenses resulting from unexpected complications due to allergic reactions or interactions among medications.

Earnings: Median annual wage and salary earnings of pharmacists in May 2004 were $84,900. The middle 50 percent earned between $75,720 and $94,850 a year. The lowest 10 percent earned less than $61,200 and the highest 10 percent earned more than $109,850 a year. Median annual earnings in the industries employing the largest numbers of pharmacists in May 2004 were:

Department stores	$86,720
Grocery stores	85,680
Health and personal care stores	85,380
General medical and surgical hospitals	84,560
Other general merchandise stores	84,170

Pharmacy Aides

Significant Points: Job opportunities are expected to be good for full-time and part-time work, especially for those with related work experience.

Many pharmacy aides work evenings, weekends and holidays.

About 80 percent work in retail pharmacies, grocery stores, department stores, or mass retailers.

Nature of the Work: Pharmacy aides help licensed pharmacists with administrative duties in running a pharmacy. Aides often are clerks or cashiers who primarily answer telephones, handle money, stock shelves and perform other clerical duties.

They work closely with pharmacy technicians. *Pharmacy technicians* usually perform more complex tasks than do aides, although in some States the duties and titles of the jobs overlap. Aides refer any questions regarding prescriptions, drug information, or health matters to a pharmacist.

Aides have several important duties that help the pharmacy to function smoothly. They may establish and maintain patient profiles, prepare insurance claim forms and stock and take inventory of prescription and over-the-counter medications. Accurate record-keeping is necessary to help avert dangerous drug interactions. In addition, because many people have medical insurance to help pay for prescriptions, it is essential that pharmacy aides correspond efficiently and correctly with the third-party insurance providers to obtain payment. Pharmacy aides also maintain inventory and inform the supervisor of stock needs so that the pharmacy does not run out of the vital medications that customers need. Some also clean pharmacy equipment, help with the maintenance of equipment and supplies and manage the cash register.

Working Conditions: Pharmacy aides work in clean, organized, well-lighted and well-ventilated areas. Most of their workday is spent on their feet. They may be required to lift heavy boxes or to use stepladders to retrieve supplies from high shelves.

Aides work the same hours that pharmacists work. These include evenings, nights, weekends and some holidays, particularly in facilities, such as hospitals and retail pharmacies that are open 24 hours a day. There are many opportunities for part-time work in both retail and hospital settings.

Training, Other Qualifications and Advancement: Most pharmacy aides receive informal on-the-job training, but employers favour those with at least a high school diploma. Prospective pharmacy aides with experience working as cashiers may have an advantage when applying for jobs. Employers also prefer applicants with strong customer service and communication skills, experience managing inventories and experience using computers. Aides entering the field need strong spelling, reading and mathematics skills.

Successful pharmacy aides are organized, dedicated, friendly and responsible. They should be willing and able to take directions. Candidates interested in becoming pharmacy aides cannot have prior records of drug or substance abuse. Strong interpersonal and communication skills are needed because pharmacy aides interact daily with patients, coworkers and health care professionals. Teamwork is very important because aides are often required to work with technicians and pharmacists.

Pharmacy aides almost always are trained on the job. They may begin by observing a more experienced worker. After they become familiar with the store's equipment, policies and procedures, they begin to work on their own. Once they become experienced, aides are not likely to receive additional training, except when new equipment is introduced or when policies or procedures change.

To become a pharmacy aide, one should be able to perform repetitive work accurately. Aides need good basic mathematics skills and good manual dexterity. Pharmacy aides should be neat in appearance and able to deal pleasantly and tactfully with customers. Some employers may prefer people with experience typing, handling money, or operating specialized equipment, including computers.

Advancement usually is limited, although some aides may decide to become pharmacy technicians or to enrol in pharmacy school to become pharmacists.

Employment: Pharmacy aides held about 50,000 jobs in 2004. About 80 percent work in retail pharmacies either independently owned or part of a drug store chain, grocery store, department store, or mass retailer; the vast majority of these are in drug stores. About 10 percent work in hospitals and the rest work in mail-order pharmacies, clinics and pharmaceutical wholesalers.

Job Outlook: Job opportunities for full-time and part-time work are expected to be good, especially for aides with related work experience in pharmacies or as cashiers or stock clerks in other retail settings. Job openings will be created by employment growth and by the need to replace workers who transfer to other occupations or leave the labour force.

Employment of pharmacy aides is expected to grow about as fast as the average for all occupations through 2014 because of the increasing use of medication in treating patients. In addition, a greater number of middle-aged and elderly people—who use more prescription drugs than younger people—will spur demand for aides in all practice settings.

Cost-conscious insurers, pharmacies and health systems will continue to employ aides. As a result, pharmacy aides will assume some responsibility for routine tasks previously performed by pharmacists and pharmacy technicians, thereby giving pharmacists more time to interact with patients and technicians more time to prepare medications. Employment of pharmacy aides will not grow as fast as employment of pharmacists and pharmacy technicians, however, because of legal limitations regarding aides' duties. Many smaller pharmacies that can afford only a small staff will favour pharmacy technicians because of their more extensive training and job skills.

Earnings: Median hourly wage and salary earnings of pharmacy aides were $8.86 in May 2004.

The middle 50 percent earned between $7.39 and $10.96; the lowest 10 percent earned less than $6.34 and the highest 10 percent earned more than $13.79. In May 2004, median hourly earnings of pharmacy aides were $8.29 in health and personal care stores and $9.80 in grocery stores.

Pharmacy Technicians

Significant Points: Job opportunities are expected to be good for full-time and part-time work, especially for those with certification or previous work experience.

Many technicians work evenings, weekends and holidays.

About 7 out of 10 of jobs were in retail pharmacies, grocery stores, department stores, or mass retailers.

Nature of the Work: Pharmacy technicians help licensed pharmacists provide medication and other health care products to patients.

Technicians usually perform routine tasks to help prepare prescribed medication for patients, such as counting tablets and labelling bottles. Technicians refer any questions regarding prescriptions, drug information, or health matters to a *pharmacist*

Pharmacy aides work closely with pharmacy technicians. They often are clerks or cashiers who primarily answer telephones, handle money, stock shelves and perform other clerical duties. Pharmacy technicians usually perform more complex tasks than do pharmacy aides, although in some States their duties and job titles may overlap.

Pharmacy technicians who work in retail or mail-order pharmacies have varying responsibilities, depending on State rules and regulations. Technicians receive written prescriptions or requests for prescription refills from patients. They also may receive prescriptions sent electronically from the doctor's office. They must verify that the information on the prescription is complete and accurate. To prepare the prescription, technicians must retrieve, count, pour, weigh, measure and sometimes mix the medication.

Then, they prepare the prescription labels, select the type of prescription container and affix the prescription and auxiliary labels to the container. Once the prescription is filled, technicians price and file the prescription, which must be checked by a pharmacist before it is given to the patient. Technicians may establish and maintain patient profiles, prepare insurance claim forms and stock and take inventory of prescription and over-the-counter medications.

In hospitals, nursing homes and assisted-living facilities, technicians have added responsibilities, including reading patients' charts and preparing and delivering the medicine to patients. Still, the pharmacist must check the order before it is delivered to the patient.

The technician then copies the information about the prescribed medication onto the patient's profile. Technicians also may assemble a 24-hour supply of medicine for every patient. They package and label each dose separately. The packages are then placed in the medicine cabinets of patients until the supervising pharmacist checks them for accuracy. The packages are then given to the patients.

Working Conditions: Pharmacy technicians work in clean, organized, well-lighted and well-ventilated areas. Most of their workday is spent on their feet. They may be required to lift heavy boxes or to use stepladders to retrieve supplies from high shelves.

Technicians work the same hours that pharmacists work. These may include evenings, nights, weekends and holidays, particularly in facilities, such as hospitals and retail pharmacies, that are open 24 hours a day. As their seniority increases, technicians often acquire increased control over the hours they work. There are many opportunities for part-time work in both retail and hospital settings.

Training, Other Qualifications and Advancement: Although most pharmacy technicians receive informal on-the-job training, employers favour those who have completed formal training and certification. However, there are currently few State and no Federal requirements for formal training or certification of pharmacy technicians. Employers who have insufficient resources to give on-the-job training often seek formally educated pharmacy technicians. Formal education programmes and certification emphasize the technician's interest in and dedication to the work. In addition to the military, some hospitals, proprietary schools, vocational or technical colleges and community colleges offer formal education programmes.

Formal pharmacy technician education programmes require classroom and laboratory work in a variety of areas, including medical and pharmaceutical terminology, pharmaceutical calculations, pharmacy record-keeping, pharmaceutical techniques and pharmacy law and ethics. Technicians also are required to learn medication names, actions, uses and doses. Many training programmes include internships, in which students gain hands-on experience in actual pharmacies. Students receive a diploma, a certificate, or an associate's degree, depending on the programme.

Prospective pharmacy technicians with experience working as an aide in a community pharmacy or volunteering in a hospital may have an advantage. Employers also prefer applicants with strong customer service and communication skills, as well as those with experience managing inventories, counting tablets, measuring dosages and using computers. Technicians entering the field need strong mathematics, spelling and reading skills. A background in chemistry, English and health education also may be beneficial. Some technicians are hired without formal training, but under the condition that they obtain certification within a specified period to retain their employment.

The Pharmacy Technician Certification Board administers the National Pharmacy Technician Certification Examination. This exam is voluntary in most States and displays the competency of the individual to act as a pharmacy technician. However, more States and employers are requiring certification as reliance on pharmacy technicians grows. Eligible candidates must have a high school diploma or GED and no felony convictions and those who pass the exam earn the title of Certified Pharmacy Technician (CPhT). The exam is offered several times per year at various locations nationally. Employers—often pharmacists—know that individuals who pass the exam have a standardized body of knowledge and skills. Many employers also will reimburse the costs of the exam as an incentive for certification.

Certified technicians must be recertified every 2 years. Technicians must complete 20 contact hours of pharmacy-related topics within the 2-year certification period to become eligible for recertification. Contact hours are awarded for on-the-job training, attending lectures and college coursework. At least 1 contact hour must be in pharmacy law. Contact hours can be earned from several different sources, including pharmacy associations, pharmacy colleges and pharmacy technician training programmes. Up to 10 contact hours can be earned when the technician is employed under the direct supervision and instruction of a pharmacist.

Successful pharmacy technicians are alert, observant, organized, dedicated and responsible. They should be willing and able to take directions. They must be precise; details are sometimes a matter of life and death. Although a pharmacist must check and approve all their work, they should be able to work independently without constant instruction from the pharmacist. Candidates interested in becoming pharmacy technicians cannot have prior records of drug or substance abuse.

Strong interpersonal and communication skills are needed because pharmacy technicians interact daily with patients, coworkers and health care professionals. Teamwork is very important because technicians often are required to work with pharmacists, aides and other technicians.

Employment: Pharmacy technicians held about 258,000 jobs in 2004. About 7 out of 10 jobs were in retail pharmacies, either independently owned or part of a drugstore chain, grocery store, department store, or mass retailer. About 2 out of 10 jobs were in hospitals and a small proportion was in mail-order and Internet pharmacies, clinics, pharmaceutical wholesalers and the Federal Government.

Job Outlook: Good job opportunities are expected for full-time and part-time work, especially for technicians with formal training or previous experience. Job openings for pharmacy technicians will result from the expansion of retaii pharmacies and other employment settings and from the need to replace workers who transfer to other occupations or leave the labour force. Employment of pharmacy technicians is expected to grow much faster than the average for all occupations through 2014 because as the population grows and ages, demand for pharmaceuticals will increase dramatically. The increased number of middle-aged and elderly people—who use more prescription drugs than younger people—will spur demand for technicians in all practice settings. With advances in science, more medications are becoming available to treat a greater number of conditions.

In addition, cost-conscious insurers, pharmacies and health systems will continue to expand the role of technicians. As a result, pharmacy technicians will assume responsibility for some of the more routine tasks previously performed by pharmacists. Pharmacy technicians also will need to learn and master new pharmacy technology as it emerges. For example, robotic machines are being increasingly used to dispense medicine into containers; technicians must oversee the machines, stock the bins and label the containers. Thus, while automation is increasingly incorporated into the job, it will not necessarily reduce the need for technicians.

Almost all States have legislated the maximum number of technicians who can safely work under a pharmacist at one time. In some States, technicians have assumed more medication-dispensing duties as pharmacists have become more involved in patient care, resulting in more technicians per pharmacist. Changes in these laws could directly affect employment.

Earnings: Median hourly earnings of wage and salary pharmacy technicians in May 2004 were $11.37. The middle 50 percent earned between $9.40 and $13.85. The lowest 10 percent earned less than $7.96 and the highest 10 percent earned more than $16.61. Median hourly earnings in the industries employing the largest numbers of pharmacy technicians in May 2004 were:

General medical and surgical hospitals	$12.93
Grocery stores	11.77
Other general merchandise stores	11.11
Department stores	10.56
Health and personal care stores	10.51

Certified technicians may earn more. Shift differentials for working evenings or weekends also can increase earnings. Some technicians belong to unions representing hospital or grocery store workers.

Psychology

Psychology can be broadly defined as the study of the mind. To pursue this career, one has to have a genuine interest in people. As a science, it is a systematic approach to the understanding of people and their behaviour. As a profession, it is the application of the understanding of human behaviour to help solve human problems.

Since psychology deals with human behaviour, psychologists apply their knowledge and techniques to a wide range of human services, management, education, law and sports.

Psychologists gather information through controlled laboratory experiments, personality, performance, aptitude and intelligence tests; observation, interviews and questionnaires, clinical studies and surveys. In addition to the variety of work settings, psychologists specialise in many different areas.

Physicians and Surgeons

Significant Points: Many physicians and surgeons work long, irregular hours; over one-third of full-time physicians worked 60 or more hours a week in 2004.

Formal education and training requirements are among the most demanding of any occupation, but earnings are among the highest.

Job opportunities should be very good, particularly in rural and low-income areas.

New physicians are much less likely to enter solo practice and more likely to work as salaried employees of group medical practices, clinics, hospitals, or health networks.

Nature of the Work: Physicians and surgeons serve a fundamental role in our society and have an effect upon all our lives. They diagnose illnesses and prescribe and administer treatment for people suffering from injury or disease. Physicians examine patients, obtain medical histories and order, perform and interpret diagnostic tests. They counsel patients on diet, hygiene and preventive health care.

There are two types of physicians: M.D.—Doctor of Medicine—and D.O.—Doctor of Osteopathic Medicine. M.D.s also are known as allopathic physicians. While both M.D.s and D.O.s may use all accepted methods of treatment, including drugs and surgery, D.O.s place special emphasis on the body's musculoskeletal system, preventive medicine and holistic patient care. D.O.s are more likely than M.D.s to be primary care specialists although they can be found in all specialities. About half of D.O.s practice general or family medicine, general internal medicine, or general pediatrics.

Physicians work in one or more of several specialities, including, but not limited to, anesthesiology, family and general medicine, general internal medicine, general pediatrics, obstetrics and gynecology, psychiatry and surgery.

***Anesthesiologists*:** Anesthesiologists focus on the care of surgical patients and pain relief. Like other physicians, they evaluate and treat patients and direct the efforts of those on their staffs. Anesthesiologists confer with other physicians and surgeons about appropriate treatments and procedures before, during and after operations. These critical care specialists are responsible for maintenance of the patient's vital life functions—heart rate, body temperature, blood pressure, breathing—

through continual monitoring and assessment during surgery. They often work outside of the operating room, providing pain relief in the intensive care unit, during labour and delivery and for those who suffer from chronic pain.

***Family and General Practitioners*:** Family and general practitioners are often the first point of contact for people seeking health care, acting as the traditional family doctor. They assess and treat a wide range of conditions, ailments and injuries, from sinus and respiratory infections to broken bones and scrapes. Family and general practitioners typically have a patient base of regular, long-term visitors. Patients with more serious conditions are referred to specialists or other health care facilities for more intensive care.

***General Internists*:** General internists diagnose and provide nonsurgical treatment for diseases and injuries of internal organ systems. They provide care mainly for adults who have a wide range of problems associated with the internal organs, such as the stomach, kidneys, liver and digestive tract. Internists use a variety of diagnostic techniques to treat patients through medication or hospitalization. Like general practitioners, general internists are commonly looked upon as primary care specialists. They have patients referred to them by other specialists, in turn referring patients to those and yet other specialists when more complex care is required.

***General Pediatricians*:** Providing care from birth to early adulthood, pediatricians are concerned with the health of infants, children and teenagers. They specialize in the diagnosis and treatment of a variety of ailments specific to young people and track their patients' growth to adulthood. Like most physicians, pediatricians work with different health care workers, such as nurses and other physicians, to assess and treat children with various ailments, such as muscular dystrophy. Most of the work of pediatricians, however, involves treating day-to-day illnesses that are common to children—minor injuries, infectious diseases and immunizations—much as a general practitioner treats adults. Some pediatricians specialize in serious medical conditions and pediatric surgery, treating auto immune disorders or serious chronic ailments.

***Obstetricians and Gynecologists*:** Obstetricians and gynecologists (ob/gyns) are specialists whose focus is women's health. They are responsible for general medical care for women, but also provide care related to pregnancy and the reproductive system.

Like general practitioners, ob/gyns are concerned with the prevention, diagnosis and treatment of general health problems, but they focus on ailments specific to the female anatomy, such as breast and cervical cancer, urinary tract and pelvic disorders and hormonal disorders. Ob/gyns also specialize in childbirth, treating and counselling women throughout their pregnancy, from giving prenatal diagnoses to delivery and postpartum care. Ob/gyns track the health of and treat, both mother and fetus as the pregnancy progresses.

***Psychiatrists*:** Psychiatrists are the primary caregivers in the area of mental health. They assess and treat mental illnesses through a combination of psychotherapy, psychoanalysis, hospitalization and medication. Psychotherapy involves regular discussions with patients about their problems; the psychiatrist helps them find solutions through changes in their behavioural patterns, the exploration of their past experiences and group and family therapy sessions.

Psychoanalysis involves long-term psychotherapy and counselling for patients. In many cases, medications are administered to correct chemical imbalances that may be causing emotional problems. Psychiatrists may also administer electroconvulsive therapy to those of their patients who do not respond to, or who cannot take, medications.

***Surgeons*:** Surgeons are physicians who specialize in the treatment of injury, disease and deformity through operations. Using a variety of instruments and with patients under general or local anesthesia, a surgeon corrects physical deformities, repairs bone and tissue after injuries, or performs preventive surgeries on patients with debilitating diseases or disorders.

Although a large number perform general surgery, many surgeons choose to specialize in a specific area. One of the most prevalent specialities is orthopedic surgery: the treatment of the musculoskeletal system. Others include neurological surgery (treatment of the brain and nervous system), cardiovascular surgery, otolaryngology (treatment of the ear, nose and throat) and plastic or reconstructive surgery. Like primary care and other specialist physicians, surgeons also examine patients, perform and interpret diagnostic tests and counsel patients on preventive health care.

A number of other medical and surgical specialists, including allergists, cardiologists, dermatologists, emergency physicians, gastroenterologists, ophthalmologists, pathologists and radiologists, also work in clinics, hospitals and private offices.

Working Conditions: Many physicians—primarily general and family practitioners, general internists, pediatricians, ob/gyns and psychiatrists—work in small private offices or clinics, often assisted by a small staff of nurses and other administrative personnel. Increasingly, physicians are practicing in groups or health care organizations that provide backup coverage and allow for more time off. These physicians often work as part of a team coordinating care for a population of patients; they are less independent than solo practitioners of the past.

Surgeons and anesthesiologists typically work in well-lighted, sterile environments while performing surgery and often stand for long periods. Most work in hospitals or in surgical outpatient centres. Many physicians and surgeons work long, irregular hours. Over one-third of full-time physicians and surgeons worked 60 hours or more a week in 2004. Only 8 percent of all physicians and surgeons worked part-time, compared with 16 percent for all occupations. Physicians and surgeons must travel frequently between office and hospital to care for their patients. Those who are on call deal with many patients' concerns over the phone and may make emergency visits to hospitals or nursing homes.

Training, Other Qualifications and Advancement: Formal education and training requirements for physicians are among the most demanding of any occupation—4 years of undergraduate school, 4 years of medical school and 3 to 8 years of internship and residency, depending on the speciality selected. A few medical schools offer combined undergraduate and medical school programmes that last 6 rather than the customary 8 years.

Premedical students must complete undergraduate work in physics, biology, mathematics, English and inorganic and organic chemistry. Students also take courses in the humanities and the social sciences. Some students volunteer at local hospitals or clinics to gain practical experience in the health professions.

The minimum educational requirement for entry into a medical school is 3 years of college; most applicants, however, have at least a bachelor's degree and many have advanced degrees. There are 146 medical schools in the United States—126 teach allopathic medicine and award a Doctor of Medicine (M.D.) degree; 20 teach osteopathic medicine and award the Doctor of Osteopathic Medicine (D.O.) degree. Acceptance to medical school is highly competitive. Applicants must submit transcripts, scores from the Medical College Admission Test and letters of recommendation. Schools also consider an applicant's character, personality, leadership qualities and participation in extracurricular activities. Most schools require an interview with members of the admissions committee.

Students spend most of the first 2 years of medical school in laboratories and classrooms, taking courses such as anatomy, biochemistry, physiology, pharmacology, psychology, microbiology, pathology, medical ethics and laws governing medicine. They also learn to take medical histories, examine patients and diagnose illnesses. During their last 2 years, students work with patients under the supervision of experienced physicians in hospitals and clinics, learning acute, chronic, preventive and rehabilitative care. Through rotations in internal medicine, family practice, obstetrics and gynecology, pediatrics, psychiatry and surgery, they gain experience in the diagnosis and treatment of illness.

Following medical school, almost all M.D.s enter a residency—graduate medical education in a speciality that takes the form of paid on-the-job training, usually in a hospital. Most D.O.s serve a 12-month rotating internship after graduation and before entering a residency, which may last 2 to 6 years.

All States, the District of Columbia and U.S. territories license physicians. To be licensed, physicians must graduate from an accredited medical school, pass a licensing examination and complete 1 to 7 years of graduate medical education. Although physicians licensed in one State usually can get a license to practice in another without further examination, some States limit reciprocity. Graduates of foreign medical schools generally can qualify for licensure after passing an examination and completing a U.S. residency.

M.D.s and D.O.s seeking board certification in a speciality may spend up to 7 years in residency training, depending on the speciality. A final examination immediately after residency or after 1 or 2 years of practice also is necessary for certification by a member board of the American Board of Medical Specialists (ABMS) or the American Osteopathic Association (AOA). The ABMS represents 24 speciality boards, ranging from allergy and immunology to urology. The AOA has approved 18 speciality boards, ranging from anesthesiology to surgery. For certification in a subspecialty, physicians usually need another 1 to 2 years of residency.

A physician's training is costly. According to the Association of American Medical Colleges, in 2004 more than 80 percent of medical school graduates were in debt for educational expenses.

People who wish to become physicians must have a desire to serve patients, be self-motivated and be able to survive the pressures and long hours of medical education and practice. Physicians also must have a good bedside manner, emotional stability and the ability to make decisions in emergencies. Prospective physicians must be willing to study throughout their career in order to keep up with medical advances.

Employment: Physicians and surgeons held about 567,000 jobs in 2004; approximately 1 out of 7 was self-employed and not incorporated. About 60 percent of salaried physicians and surgeons were in office of physicians and 16 percent were employed by private hospitals. Others practiced in Federal, State and local governments, including hospitals, colleges, universities and professional schools; private colleges, universities and professional schools; and outpatient care centres.

According to the American Medical Association (AMA), in 2003 about 2 out 5 physicians in patient care were in primary care, but not in a subspecialty of primary care.

Percent Distribution of Physicians by Speciality

Percent	*Total*
100.0	Primary care
40.8	Family medicine and general practice
12.8	Internal medicine
15.1	Obstetrics & gynecology
5.3	Pediatrics
7.6	Specialities
59.2	Anesthesiology
5.4	Psychiatry
5.4	Surgical specialities, selected
14.6	All other specialities

Source: American Medical Association, Physician Characteristics and Distribution in the US, 2005.

A growing number of physicians are partners or salaried employees of group practices. Organized as clinics or as associations of physicians, medical groups can afford expensive medical equipment and realize other business advantages.

According to the AMA, the New England and Middle Atlantic States have the highest ratio of physicians to population; the South Central and Mountain States have the lowest. D.O.s are more likely than M.D.s to practice in small cities and towns and in rural areas. M.D.s tend to locate in urban areas, close to hospital and education centres.

Job Outlook: Employment of physicians and surgeons is projected to grow faster than average for all occupations through the year 2014 due to continued expansion of health care industries. The growing and aging population will drive overall growth in the demand for physician services, as consumers continue to demand high levels of care using the latest technologies, diagnostic tests and therapies. In addition to employment growth, job openings will result from the need to replace physicians and surgeons who retire over the 2004-14 period.

Demand for physicians' services is highly sensitive to changes in consumer preferences, health care reimbursement policies and legislation. For example, if changes to health coverage result in consumers facing higher out-of-pocket costs, they may demand fewer physician services.

Demand for physician services may also be tempered by patients relying more on other health care providers—such as physician assistants, nurse practitioners, optometrists and nurse anesthetists—for some health care services. In addition, new technologies will increase physician productivity. Telemedicine will allow physicians to treat patients or consult with other providers remotely. Increasing use of electronic medical records, test and prescription orders, billing and scheduling will also improve physician productivity.

Opportunities for individuals interested in becoming physicians and surgeons are expected to be very good. Reports of shortages in some specialities or geographic areas should attract new entrants, encouraging schools to expand programmes and hospitals to expand available residency slots. However, because physician training is so lengthy, employment change happens gradually.

In the short term, to meet increased demand, experienced physicians may work longer hours, delay retirement, or take measures to increase productivity, such as using more support staff to provide services. Opportunities should be particularly good in rural and low-income areas, because some physicians find these areas unattractive due to less control over work hours, isolation from medical colleagues, or other reasons.

Unlike their predecessors, newly trained physicians face radically different choices of where and how to practice. New physicians are much less likely to enter solo practice and more likely to take salaried jobs in group medical practices, clinics and health networks.

Earnings: Earnings of physicians and surgeons are among the highest of any occupation. According to the Medical Group Management Association's Physician Compensation and Production Survey, median total compensation for physicians in 2004 varied by speciality, as shown in table. Total compensation for physicians reflects the amount reported as direct compensation for tax purposes, plus all voluntary salary reductions. Salary, bonus and/or incentive payments, research stipends, honoraria and distribution of profits were included in total compensation.

Median Total Compensation of Physicians by Speciality

Less than two years in speciality	*Over one year in speciality*	
Anesthesiology	$259,948	$321,686
Surgery: General	228,839	282,504
Obstetrics/gynecology: General	203,270	247,348
Psychiatry: General	173,922	180,000
Internal medicine: General	141,912	166,420
Pediatrics: General	132,953	161,331
Family practice (without obstetrics)	137,119	156,010

Source: Medical Group Management Association, Physician Compensation and Production Report, 2005.

Self-employed physicians—those who own or are part owners of their medical practice—generally have higher median incomes than salaried physicians. Earnings vary according to number of years in practice, geographic region, hours worked and skill, personality and professional reputation. Self-employed physicians and surgeons must provide for their own health insurance and retirement.

Veterinary Science

Do you fight for the cause of the neighbourhood mongrels? Do you feed them scraps of leftovers and act as a referee in their fights amongst themselves? Were you always the one to pick up injured pigeons and keep them well-fed and warm till they recovered? If you were the one to do all, or any of these, you might have it in you to be a vet, so it's time you gave it a serious thought.

Veterinary science offers a large number of avenues of work. Besides regular practice, vets can also take up research work, either on their own or in association with the government. Opportunities also abound in livestock management.

Being a vet does not only mean being fond of animals; it also means the ability to empathise with their needs, to be able to locate their specific problems and communicate to them the fact that you are trying to help them. Building and maintaining a special bond between yourself and the animal you are going to treat is very important, as animals are unfailingly sensitive towards the people who deal with them (or people they have to deal with, whichever way you prefer to look at it!). An inherent respect for them is as important as being sympathetic towards their suffering. They do not like condescension any more than you do or I do, believe me!

Here we have complete and comprehensive information on veterinary science as a career. From how to go about making a career in this field to institutes offering courses, we tell you all. All that's left for you to do is follow it and there, you might be another Dr. Doolittle in the making!

Veterinary Technologists and Technicians

Significant Points: Animal lovers get satisfaction in this occupation, but aspects of the work can be unpleasant, physically and emotionally demanding and sometimes dangerous.

Entrants generally complete a 2-year or 4-year veterinary technology programme and must pass a State examination.

Employment is expected to grow much faster than average.

Keen competition is expected for jobs in zoos.

Nature of the Work: Owners of pets and other animals today expect state-of-the-art veterinary care. To provide this service, veterinarians use the skills of veterinary technologists and technicians, who perform many of the same duties for a veterinarian that a nurse would for a physician, including routine laboratory and clinical procedures. Although specific job duties vary by employer, there often is little difference between the tasks carried out by technicians and by technologists, despite some differences in formal education and training. As a result, most workers in this occupation are called technicians.

Veterinary technologists and technicians typically conduct clinical work in a private practice under the supervision of a veterinarian—often performing various medical tests along with treating and diagnosing medical conditions and diseases in animals. For example, they may perform laboratory tests such as urinalysis and blood counts, assist with dental prophylaxis, prepare tissue samples, take blood samples, or assist veterinarians in a variety of tests and analyses in which they often utilize various items of medical equipment, such as test tubes and diagnostic equipment.

While most of these duties are performed in a laboratory setting, many are not. For example, some veterinary technicians obtain and record patients' case histories, expose and develop x rays and provide specialized nursing care. In addition, experienced veterinary technicians may discuss a pet's condition with its owners and train new clinic personnel. Veterinary technologists and technicians assisting small-animal practitioners usually care for companion animals, such as cats and dogs, but can perform a variety of duties with mice, rats, sheep, pigs, cattle, monkeys, birds, fish and frogs. Very few veterinary technologists work in mixed animal practices where they care for both small companion animals and larger, nondomestic animals.

Besides working in private clinics and animal hospitals, veterinary technologists and technicians may work in research facilities, where they may administer medications orally or topically, prepare samples for laboratory examinations and record information on an animal's genealogy, diet, weight, medications, food intake and clinical signs of pain and distress. Some may be required to sterilize laboratory and surgical equipment and provide routine postoperative care. At research facilities, veterinary technologists typically work under the guidance of veterinarians, physicians and other laboratory technicians. Some veterinary technologists vaccinate newly admitted animals and occasionally are required to euthanize seriously ill, severely injured, or unwanted animals. While the goal of most veterinary technologists and technicians is to promote animal health, some contribute to human health as well.

Veterinary technologists occasionally assist veterinarians as they work with other scientists in medical-related fields such as gene therapy and cloning. Some find opportunities in biomedical research, wildlife medicine, the military, livestock management, or pharmaceutical sales.

Working Conditions: People who love animals get satisfaction from working with and helping them. However, some of the work may be unpleasant, physically and emotionally demanding and sometimes dangerous. At times, veterinary technicians must clean cages and lift, hold, or restrain animals, risking exposure to bites or scratches. These workers must take precautions when treating animals with germicides or insecticides. The work setting can be noisy.

Veterinary technologists and technicians who witness abused animals or who euthanize unwanted, aged, or hopelessly injured animals may experience emotional stress. Those working for humane societies and animal shelters often deal with the public, some of whom might react with hostility to any implication that the owners are neglecting or abusing their pets. Such workers must maintain a calm and professional demeanour while they enforce the laws regarding animal care. In some animal hospitals, research facilities and animal shelters, a veterinary technician is on duty 24 hours a day, which means that some may work night shifts. Most full-time veterinary technologists and technicians work about 40 hours a week, although some work 50 or more hours a week.

Training, Other Qualifications and Advancement: There are primarily two levels of education and training for entry to this occupation: a 2-year programme for veterinary technicians and a 4-year programme for veterinary technologists. Most entry-level veterinary technicians have a 2-year degree, usually an associate's degree, from an accredited community college programme in veterinary technology in which courses are taught in clinical and laboratory settings using live animals. About 15 colleges offer veterinary technology programmes that are longer and that culminate in a 4-year bachelor's degree in veterinary technology. These 4-year colleges, in addition to some vocational schools, also offer 2-year programmes in laboratory animal science. Approximately 5 schools offer distance learning.

In 2004, 116 veterinary technology programmes in 43 States were accredited by the American Veterinary Medical Association (AVMA). Graduation from an AVMA-accredited veterinary technology programme allows students to take the credentialing exam in any State in the country. Each State regulates veterinary technicians and technologists differently; however, all States require them to pass a credentialing exam following coursework.

Passing the State exam assures the public that the technician or technologist has sufficient knowledge to work in a veterinary clinic or hospital. Candidates are tested for competency through an examination that includes oral, written and practical portions and that is regulated by the State Board of Veterinary Examiners or the appropriate State agency. Depending on the State, candidates may become registered, licensed, or certified. Most States, however, use the National Veterinary Technician (NVT) exam. Prospects usually can have their passing scores transferred from one State to another, so long as both States utilize the same exam.

Employers recommend American Association for Laboratory Animal Science (AALAS) certification for those seeking employment in a research facility. AALAS offers certification for three levels of technician competence, with a focus on three principal areas—animal husbandry, facility management and animal health and welfare.

Those who wish to become certified must satisfy a combination of education and experience requirements prior to taking an exam. Work experience must be directly related to the maintenance, health and well-being of laboratory animals and must be gained in a laboratory animal facility as defined by AALAS. Candidates who meet the necessary criteria can begin pursuing the desired certification on the basis of their qualifications. The lowest level of certification is Assistant Laboratory Animal Technician (ALAT), the second level is Laboratory Animal Technician (LAT) and the highest level of certification is Laboratory Animal Technologist (LATG). The examination consists of multiple-choice questions and is longer and more difficult for higher levels of certification, ranging from 2 hours for the ALAT to 3 hours for the LATG.

Persons interested in careers as veterinary technologists and technicians should take as many high school science, biology and math courses as possible. Science courses taken beyond high school, in an associate's or bachelor's degree programme, should emphasize practical skills in a clinical or laboratory setting. Because veterinary technologists and technicians often deal with pet owners, communication skills are very important. In addition, technologists and technicians should be able to work well with others, because teamwork with veterinarians is common. Organizational ability and the ability to pay attention to detail also are important.

Technologists and technicians usually begin work as trainees in routine positions under the direct supervision of a veterinarian. Entry-level workers whose training or educational background encompasses extensive hands-on experience with a variety of laboratory equipment, including diagnostic and medical equipment, usually require a shorter period of on-the-job training. As they gain experience, technologists and technicians take on more responsibility and carry out more assignments under only general veterinary supervision. Some eventually may become supervisors.

Employment: Veterinary technologists and technicians held about 60,000 jobs in 2004. Most worked in veterinary services. The remainder worked in boarding kennels, animal shelters, stables, grooming salons, zoos and local, State and Federal agencies.

Job Outlook: Employment of veterinary technologists and technicians is expected to grow much faster than average for all occupations through the year 2014. Job openings also will stem from the need to replace veterinary technologists and technicians who leave the occupation over the 2004–14 period.

Keen competition is expected for veterinary technologist and technician jobs in zoos, due to expected slow growth in zoo capacity, low turnover among workers, the limited number of positions and the fact that the occupation attracts many candidates.

Pet owners are becoming more affluent and more willing to pay for advanced care because many of them consider their pet to be part of the family. This growing affluence and view of pets will spur employment growth for veterinary technologists and technicians.

The number of dogs used as companion pets, which also drives employment growth, is expected to increase more slowly during the projection period than in the previous decade. However, the rapidly growing number of cats utilized as companion pets is expected to boost the demand for feline medicine and services, offsetting any reduced demand for veterinary care for dogs.

The availability of advanced veterinary services, such as preventive dental care and surgical procedures, may provide opportunities for workers specializing in those areas. Biomedical facilities, diagnostic laboratories, wildlife facilities, humane societies, animal control facilities, drug or food manufacturing companies and food safety inspection facilities will provide additional jobs for veterinary technologists and technicians. Furthermore, demand for these workers will stem from the desire to replace veterinary assistants with more highly skilled technicians and technologists in animal clinics and hospitals, shelters, kennels and humane societies.

Employment of veterinary technicians and technologists is relatively stable during periods of economic recession. Layoffs are less likely to occur among veterinary technologists and technicians than in some other occupations because animals will continue to require medical care.

Earnings: Median hourly earnings of veterinary technologists and technicians were $11.99 in May 2004. The middle 50 percent earned between $9.88 and $14.56. The bottom 10 percent earned less than $8.51 and the top 10 percent earned more than $17.12.

Nursing Career

Does nursing remind you of mundane bedside practices and gloomy hospital atmosphere? Then this nursing career guide will help demystify this profession, what it entails and the educational requirements needed. Apart from bedside practice, a career in nursing can encompass administrative functions such as nurse administrator and nurse educator. This informative nursing career guide gives you an insight into various aspects of the nursing vocation.

Career Assessment: Career assessment tests help you evaluate your skills so that you and your organization can help you chart out your career path and job content. Career assessment tests recognize different kinds of skills in individuals. Foundation skills are those that each employee needs—thinking, people and basic skills. Some skills are transferable; they can be used in different occupations. Employers will pay candidates for their marketable skills, ones that they can use to best advantage in the organizations.

Nursing Career Options: Today, nursing is the biggest health care profession in the U.S. with almost 2.6 million registered nurses (RN). Career opportunities are myriad and you can work in a variety of practice settings such as hospitals, long-term care facilities, community and public health agencies, independent practice, ambulatory care centres, U.S. Public Health Service, military services (Army, Navy and Air Force), Veteran's Administration Medical centres and in any setting where health care services are needed. Nursing practice areas also include childcare, including newborn infants and caring for the elderly and services for pregnant women. The operation room, critical care and emergency departments are areas where trained and specialized nurses are needed. Other speciality areas of nursing are injury nursing, cancer nursing and caring for heart attack and heart surgery.

A career in nursing offers considerable amount of flexibility. As a nurse you can either work in one setting or take short-term assignments as travel nurse. Travel nurses fill temporary assignments for nursing staff all over the globe. However nurses with advanced education become nurse practitioners, clinical nurse specialists, educators, researchers and managers. The two new areas in nursing career are tele-health nursing and overall patient care. Practicing tele-health involves expert knowledge that has to be disseminated over the telephone, computer or any other electronic media for counselling, teaching and monitoring patients via telephone, computer or other electronic means. This widens the possibilities and career opportunities in nursing.

Nursing Career Prospects: With over 100,000 vacant positions and an ever-growing need for healthcare workers, the career prospects in the nursing sector are on the increase. Once you finish your nursing school and become a registered nurse (RN) after hours of practical experience and specialized knowledge, you are eligible for employment. Possessing a RN status is more likely to ensure a future filled with rewarding experiences, unmatched opportunities and competitive salary and excellent benefits.

According to the American Nurses Association, "The average staff nurse working in all settings earns $35,212. (Hospital staff nurses reported $36,618.) Administrators earn $45,071. Instructors earn $36,896. Supervisors earn $38,979. The average Clinical Nurse Specialist earns $41,226; Nurse Practitioners on average earn $71,000, Nurse Anesthetists: $113,000." (Based on US Department of Labour's Statistics on Registered Nurses).

On an average an entry-level staff nurse may be paid $30,000 to $45,000 per year plus additional pay for evening, night and weekend shifts. There are also attractive benefit packages for nurses at all levels. These include health insurance, holiday pay, vacation, college tuition reimbursement, childcare, flexible scheduling and pension plans. However, nurse practitioners, clinical nurse specialists and nurses with advanced degrees earn considerably higher salaries. Some are eligible to receive direct payment from insurance companies for their services.

Nursing Career Guide

Entry Level Education/ Degrees: In order to become a registered nurse (RN), you need to graduate from a nursing programme. This enables you to take the state licensure examination. There are more than 1500 nursing programmes in the U.S. and there are three types of nursing programmes that prepare you to assume different roles once you graduate.

Bachelor of Science in Nursing (BS/BSN): This four-year programme offered at all colleges and universities offers considerable opportunities for career growth. Apart from independent nursing roles, BSN graduates are prepared for all health care settings including leadership and management. BSN is essential for acquiring master's degree in nursing. BSN is preferred and often required for military nursing, management, public health nursing, overseas/development nursing, forensic nursing and school nursing.

Associate Degree in Nursing (ADN): ADN is a two-to-three year programme offered at junior and community colleges. This course trains and prepares you to handle direct patient care in various settings. However you can also find some hospital nursing schools, colleges and universities offering ADN programme.

Hospital Diploma: This two-to-three year diploma programme is based in hospital settings. Many diploma schools are affiliated with junior colleges, where you may also take basic science and English requirements, thereby earning an Associate's Degree along with a diploma in nursing.

Licensure

After completing a nursing programme, you are required to pass the National Council Licensure Examination to become a Registered Nurse (NCLEX-RN). This test is taken after graduating from a state-approved nursing school. These examinations are offered through State Board of Nursing.

Advanced Degrees in Nursing: Advanced degrees in nursing help you specialize in your area of interest/focus. The advanced degree programmes vary from degree completion programmes for RNs (RNs to BSN/RN to MSN) to master's degree to doctoral and post-doctoral programmes. Hundreds of bridge programmes are offered for nurses with diplomas and ADN degrees who wish to complete a Bachelor's or Master's degree programme in nursing. Meanwhile master's degree programme prepares nurses for more independent roles such as nurse practitioner, nurse midwife, nurse anesthetist or nurse psychotherapist to name a few.

Nursing Positions: After completing your nursing programme you can take up a variety of nursing positions based on your level of education and experience.

Case Manager: Nurse Case Manager helps in the process of organizing and coordinating resources and services in response to individual health care needs.

Certified Nurse Midwife: This speciality nurse supports childbearing women during preconception, prenatal, labour and delivery and postpartum periods as well as provides family-planning counselling and gynecological care.

Staff Nurse: The entry-level staff nurse makes nursing judgments based on scientific knowledge and relies on procedures and standardized care plans.

The other nursing positions include Clinical nurse specialist, Manger/Administrator, Nurse Anesthetist, Nurse Educator and Nurse Practitioner.

Nursing Specialities

The master's programme in nursing helps you specialize in one single area and enables you to don independent nursing roles.

Radiology Nursing: Radiology nurses provide care and support to patients undergoing diagnosis in radiation imaging environments including ultrasonography, magnetic resonance and radiation oncology.

Rehabilitation Nursing: Nurses in this field provide physical and emotional support to patients and the families of patients with illnesses or disabilities that affect their ability to function normally. They aid in the patient's altered lifestyles.

AIDS Care Nursing: These nurses respond to the physical, psychological, spiritual and social concerns of patients with AIDS. They care for the chronically ill and those dying with numerous clinical manifestations.

Forensic Nursing: Nurses in this sector work with law enforcement officials to aid in the investigation of crimes such as sexual assault, accidental death, abuse and assault. They also treat the victims of these crimes.

Meanwhile nursing specialities also include Ambulatory care nursing, Genetic nursing, Gastroenterology / Endoscopy nursing, Intravenous therapy nursing, Long-term care nursing, sub acute care nursing, transplant nursing, school nursing, psychiatric nursing, orthopedic nursing, ophthalmic nursing, trauma nursing—the list is long!

You can find many nursing organizations online, providing a detailed vision of each nursing speciality, American Academy of Nursing, American Nurses Association and National Student Nurses Association being among the prominent ones.

Licensed Practical and Licensed Vocational Nurses

Significant Points: Training lasting about 1 year is available in about 1,200 State-approved programmes, mostly in vocational or technical schools.

Applicants for jobs in hospitals may face competition as the number of hospital jobs for licensed practical nurses declines; however, rapid employment growth is projected in other health care industries, with the best job opportunities occurring in nursing care facilities and in home health care services.

Replacement needs will be a major source of job openings, as many workers leave the occupation permanently.

Nature of the Work: Licensed practical nurses (LPNs), or licensed vocational nurses (LVNs), care for the sick, injured, convalescent and disabled under the direction of physicians and registered nurses.

Most LPNs provide basic bedside care, taking vital signs such as temperature, blood pressure, pulse and respiration. They also prepare and give injections and enemas, monitor catheters, apply dressings, treat bedsores and give alcohol rubs and massages. LPNs monitor their patients and report adverse reactions to medications or treatments. They collect samples for testing, perform routine laboratory tests, feed patients and record food and fluid intake and output. To help keep patients comfortable, LPNs assist with bathing, dressing and personal hygiene. In States where the law allows, they may administer prescribed medicines or start intravenous fluids. Some LPNs help to deliver, care for and feed infants. Experienced LPNs may supervise nursing assistants and aides.

In addition to providing routine bedside care, LPNs in nursing care facilities help to evaluate residents' needs, develop care plans and supervise the care provided by nursing aides. In doctors' offices and clinics, they also may make appointments, keep records and perform other clerical duties. LPNs who work in private homes may prepare meals and teach family members simple nursing tasks.

Working Conditions: Most licensed practical nurses in hospitals and nursing care facilities work a 40-hour week, but because patients need round-the-clock care, some work nights, weekends and holidays. They often stand for long periods and help patients move in bed, stand, or walk.

LPNs may face hazards from caustic chemicals, radiation and infectious diseases such as hepatitis. They are subject to back injuries when moving patients and shock from electrical equipment. They often must deal with the stress of heavy workloads. In addition, the patients they care for may be confused, irrational, agitated, or uncooperative.

Training, Other Qualifications and Advancement: All States and the District of Columbia require LPNs to pass a licensing examination, known as the NCLEX-PN, after completing a State-approved practical nursing programme. A high school diploma or its equivalent usually is required for entry, although some programmes accept candidates without a diploma and some are designed as part of a high school curriculum.

In 2004, approximately 1,200 State-approved programmes provided training in practical nursing. Most training programmes are available from technical and vocational schools, or from community and junior colleges. Other programmes are available through high schools, hospitals and colleges and universities.

Most practical nursing programmes last about 1 year and include both classroom study and supervised clinical practice (patient care). Classroom study covers basic nursing concepts and patient care-related subjects, including anatomy, physiology, medical-surgical nursing, pediatrics, obstetrics, psychiatric nursing, the administration of drugs, nutrition and first aid. Clinical practice usually is in a hospital, but sometimes includes other settings. In some employment settings, such as nursing homes, LPNs can advance to become charge nurses who oversee the work of other LPNs and of nursing aides. Some LPNs also choose to become registered nurses through numerous LPN-to-RN training programmes.

LPNs should have a caring, sympathetic nature. They should be emotionally stable because working with the sick and injured can be stressful. They also should have keen observational, decision-making and communication skills. As part of a health care team, they must be able to follow orders and work under close supervision.

Employment: Licensed practical nurses held about 726,000 jobs in 2004. About 27 percent of LPNs worked in hospitals, 25 percent in nursing care facilities and another 12 percent in offices of physicians. Others worked for home health care services; employment services; community care facilities for the elderly; public and private educational services; outpatient care centres; and Federal, State and local government agencies. About 1 in 5 worked part time.

Job Outlook: Employment of LPNs is expected to **grow about as fast as average** for all occupations through 2014 in response to the long-term care needs of an increasing elderly population and the general growth of health care services. Replacement needs will be a major source of job openings, as many workers leave the occupation permanently. Applicants for jobs in hospitals may face competition as the number of hospital jobs for LPNs declines; however, rapid employment growth is projected in other health care industries, with the best job opportunities occurring in nursing care facilities and in home health care services. Employment of LPNs in hospitals is expected to continue to decline. Sophisticated procedures once performed only in hospitals are being performed in physicians' offices and in outpatient care centres such as ambulatory surgical and emergency medical centres, largely because of advances in technology. Consequently, employment of LPNs in most health care industries outside the traditional hospital setting is projected to grow faster than average.

Employment of LPNs is expected to grow much faster than average in home health care services. Home health care agencies also will offer the most new jobs for LPNs because of an increasing number of older persons with functional disabilities, consumer preference for care in the home and technological advances that make it possible to bring increasingly complex treatments into the home.

Employment of LPNs in nursing care facilities is expected to grow about as fast as average because of the growing number of aged and disabled persons in need of long-term care. In addition, LPNs in nursing care facilities will be needed to care for the increasing number of patients who have been discharged from the hospital but who have not recovered enough to return home. However, changes in consumer preferences towards less restrictive and more cost-effective care from assisted living facilities and home health care agencies will limit employment growth.

Earnings: Median annual earnings of licensed practical nurses were $33,970 in May 2004. The middle 50 percent earned between $28,830 and $40,670. The lowest 10 percent earned less than $24,480 and the highest 10 percent earned more than $46,270. Median annual earnings in the industries employing the largest numbers of licensed practical nurses in May 2004 were:

Employment services	$41,550
Nursing care facilities	35,460
Home health care services	35,180
General medical and surgical hospitals	32,570
Offices of physicians	30,400

Nursing, Psychiatric and Home Health Aides

Significant Points: Home health aides is projected to be the fastest growing occupation through 2014.

Numerous job openings and excellent job opportunities are expected.

Most jobs are in nursing and residential care facilities, hospitals and home health care services.

Modest entry requirements, low pay, high physical and emotional demands and lack of advancement opportunities characterize this occupation.

Nature of the Work: Nursing and psychiatric aides help care for physically or mentally ill, injured, disabled, or infirm individuals confined to hospitals, nursing care facilities and mental health settings. Home health aides have duties that are similar, but they work in patients' homes or residential care facilities.

Nursing aides—also known as nursing assistants, certified nursing assistants, geriatric aides, unlicensed assistive personnel, orderlies, or hospital attendants—perform routine tasks under the supervision of nursing and medical staff. They answer patients' call lights; deliver messages; serve meals; make beds; and help patients to eat, dress and bathe. Aides also may provide skin care to patients; take their temperature, pulse rate, respiration rate and blood pressure; and help them to get into and out of bed and walk.

They also may escort patients to operating and examining rooms, keep patients' rooms neat, set up equipment, store and move supplies and assist with some procedures. Aides observe patients' physical, mental and emotional conditions and report any change to the nursing or medical staff.

Nursing aides employed in nursing care facilities often are the principal caregivers, having far more contact with residents than do other members of the staff. Because some residents may stay in a nursing care facility for months or even years, aides develop ongoing relationships with them and interact with them in a positive, caring way.

Home health aides help elderly, convalescent, or disabled persons live in their own homes instead of in a health care facility. Under the direction of nursing or medical staff, they provide health-related services, such as administering oral medications. (Personal and home care aides, who provide mainly housekeeping and routine personal care services, are discussed elsewhere in the *Handbook.*) Like nursing aides, home health aides may check patients' pulse rate, temperature and respiration rate; help with simple prescribed exercises; keep patients' rooms neat; and help patients to move from bed, bathe, dress and groom. Occasionally, they change nonsterile dressings, give massages and alcohol rubs, or assist with braces and artificial limbs. Experienced home health aides also may assist with medical equipment such as ventilators, which help patients breathe.

Most home health aides work with elderly or disabled persons who need more extensive care than family or friends can provide. Some help discharged hospital patients who have relatively short-term needs.

In home health agencies, a registered nurse, physical therapist, or social worker usually assigns specific duties to and supervises home health aides, who keep records of the services they perform and record each patient's condition and progress. The aides report changes in a patient's condition to the supervisor or case manager.

Psychiatric aides, also known as mental health assistants or psychiatric nursing assistants, care for mentally impaired or emotionally disturbed individuals. They work under a team that may include psychiatrists, psychologists, psychiatric nurses, social workers and therapists. In addition to helping patients to dress, bathe, groom themselves and eat, psychiatric aides socialize with them and lead them in educational and recreational activities. Psychiatric aides may play games such as cards with the patients, watch television with them, or participate in group activities, such as sports or field trips. They observe patients and report any physical or behavioural signs that might be important for the professional staff to know. They accompany patients to and from examinations and treatment. Because they have such close contact with patients, psychiatric aides can have a great deal of influence on their patients' outlook and treatment.

Working Conditions: Most full-time aides work about 40 hours a week, but, because patients need care 24 hours a day, some aides work evenings, nights, weekends and holidays. Many work part time. In 2004, 25 percent of aides worked part time compared with 16 percent of all workers. Aides spend many hours standing and walking and they often face heavy workloads. Aides must guard against back injury because they may have to move patients into and out of bed or help them to stand or walk. Aides also may face hazards from minor infections and major diseases, such as hepatitis, but can avoid infections by following proper procedures.

Aides often have unpleasant duties, such as emptying bedpans and changing soiled bed linens. The patients they care for may be disoriented, irritable, or uncooperative. Psychiatric aides must be prepared to care for patients whose illness may cause violent behaviour. While their work can be emotionally demanding, many aides gain satisfaction from assisting those in need.

Home health aides may go to the same patient's home for months or even years. However, most aides work with a number of different patients, each job lasting a few hours, days, or weeks. Home health aides often visit multiple patients on the same day.

Home health aides generally work alone, with periodic visits from their supervisor. They receive detailed instructions explaining when to visit patients and what services to perform. Aides are individually responsible for getting to patients' homes and they may spend a good portion of the working day travelling from one patient to another. Because mechanical lifting devices available in institutional settings are seldom available in patients' homes, home health aides are particularly susceptible to injuries resulting from overexertion when they assist patients.

Training, Other Qualifications and Advancement: In many cases, a high school diploma or equivalent is necessary for a job as a nursing or psychiatric aide. However, a high school diploma generally is not required for jobs as home health aides. Hospitals may require previous experience as a nursing aide or home health aide.

Nursing care facilities often hire inexperienced workers, who must complete a minimum of 75 hours of mandatory training and pass a competency evaluation as part of a State-approved training programme within 4 months of their employment. Aides who complete the programme are known as certified nurse assistants (CNAs) and are placed on the State registry of nursing aides. Some States also require psychiatric aides to complete a formal training programme. However, most psychiatric aides learn their skills on the job from experienced workers.

Nursing and psychiatric aide training is offered in high schools, vocational-technical centres, some nursing care facilities and some community colleges. Courses cover body mechanics, nutrition, anatomy and physiology, infection control, communication skills and resident rights. Personal care skills, such as how to help patients to bathe, eat and groom themselves, also are taught.

Some employers provide classroom instruction for newly hired aides, while others rely exclusively on informal on-the-job instruction by a licensed nurse or an experienced aide. Such training may last from several days to a few months. Aides also may attend lectures, workshops and in-service training.

The Federal Government has guidelines for home health aides whose employers receive reimbursement from Medicare. Federal law requires home health aides to pass a competency test covering a wide range of areas: communication; documentation of patient status and care provided; reading and recording of vital signs; basic infection-control procedures; basic bodily functions; maintenance of a healthy environment; emergency procedures; physical, emotional and developmental characteristics of patients; personal hygiene and grooming; safe transfer techniques; normal range of motion and positioning; and basic nutrition.

A home health aide may receive training before taking the competency test. Federal law suggests at least 75 hours of classroom and practical training, supervised by a registered nurse. Training and testing programmes may be offered by the employing agency but must meet the standards of the Centre for Medicare and Medicaid Services. State regulations for training programmes vary.

The National Association for Home Care offers national certification for home health aides. The certification is a voluntary demonstration that the individual has met industry standards. Some States also require aides to be licensed.

Aides must be in good health. A physical examination, including State-regulated tests such as those for tuberculosis, may be required. A criminal background check also is usually required for employment.

Applicants should be tactful, patient, understanding, emotionally stable and dependable and should have a desire to help people. They also should be able to work as part of a team, have good communication skills and be willing to perform repetitive, routine tasks. Home health aides should be honest and discreet, because they work in private homes. They also will need access to their own car or public transportation to reach patients' homes.

For some individuals, these occupations serve as entry-level jobs, as in the case of high school and college students who may work while also attending school. In addition, experience as an aide can help individuals decide whether to pursue a career in health care. Opportunities for advancement within these occupations are limited. Aides generally need additional formal training or education in order to enter other health occupations. The most common health care occupations for former aides are licensed practical nurse, registered nurse and medical assistant.

Employment: Nursing, psychiatric and home health aides held about 2.1 million jobs in 2004. Nursing aides held the most jobs—approximately 1.5 million. Home health aides held roughly 624,000 jobs and psychiatric aides held about 59,000 jobs. Around

42 percent of nursing aides worked in nursing care facilities and another 27 percent worked in hospitals. Most home health aides—about 34 percent—were employed by home health care services. Others were employed in nursing and residential care facilities and social assistance agencies. Around 54 percent of all psychiatric aides worked in hospitals, primarily in psychiatric and substance abuse hospitals, although some also worked in the psychiatric units of general medical and surgical hospitals. Others were employed in State government agencies; residential mental retardation, mental health and substance abuse facilities; outpatient care centres; and nursing care facilities.

Job Outlook: Numerous job openings for nursing, psychiatric and home health aides will arise from a combination of fast employment growth and high replacement needs. High replacement needs in this large occupation reflect modest entry requirements, low pay, high physical and emotional demands and lack of opportunities for advancement. For these same reasons, many people are unwilling to perform the kind of work required by the occupation, limiting the number of entrants. Many aides also leave the occupation to attend training programmes for other health care occupations. Therefore, persons who are interested in and suited for, this work should have excellent job opportunities.

Overall employment of nursing, psychiatric and home health aides is projected to grow much faster than average for all occupations through the year 2014, although individual occupational growth rates will vary. Home health aides is expected to be the fastest growing occupation, as a result of both growing demand for home services from an aging population and efforts to contain costs by moving patients out of hospitals and nursing care facilities as quickly as possible. Consumer preference for care in the home and improvements in medical technologies for in-home treatment also will contribute to much-faster-than-average employment growth for home health aides.

Nursing aide employment will not grow as fast as home health aide employment, largely because nursing aides are concentrated in slower growing nursing care facilities and hospitals. Employment of nursing aides is expected to grow faster than average for all occupations through 2014, in response to the long-term care needs of an increasing elderly population. Financial pressures on hospitals to discharge patients as soon as possible should boost admissions to nursing care facilities. As a result, job opportunities will be more numerous in nursing and residential care facilities than in hospitals. Modern medical technology also will drive demand for nursing aides because, as the technology saves and extends more lives, it increases the need for long-term care provided by aides.

Employment of psychiatric aides—the smallest of the three occupations—is expected to grow more slowly than average for all occupations. Most psychiatric aides currently work in hospitals, but most job growth will be in residential mental health facilities and in home health care agencies. There is a long-term trend toward treating mental health patients outside of hospitals because it is more cost effective and allows patients to live more normal lives. Demand for psychiatric aides in residential facilities will rise in response to growth in the number of older persons—many of whom will require mental health services—but also as an increasing number of mentally disabled adults, who were formerly cared for by their elderly parents, seek care. Job growth also could be affected by changes in government funding of programmes for the mentally ill.

Earnings: Median hourly earnings of nursing aides, orderlies and attendants were $10.09 in May 2004. The middle 50 percent earned between $8.59 and $12.09 an hour. The lowest 10 percent earned less than $7.31 and the highest 10 percent earned more than $14.02 an hour. Median hourly earnings in the industries employing the largest numbers of nursing aides, orderlies and attendants in May 2004 were as follows:

Employment services	$11.29
Local government	11.10
General medical and surgical hospitals	10.44
Nursing care facilities	9.86
Community care facilities for the elderly	9.56

Nursing and psychiatric aides in hospitals generally receive at least 1 week of paid vacation after 1 year of service. Paid holidays and sick leave, hospital and medical benefits, extra pay for late-shift work and pension plans also are available to many hospital employees and to some nursing care facility employees. Median hourly earnings of home health aides were $8.81 in May 2004. The middle 50 percent earned between $7.52 and $10.38an hour. The lowest 10 percent earned less than $6.52 and the highest 10 percent earned more than $12.32an hour. Median hourly earnings in the industries employing the largest numbers of home health aides in May 2004 were as follows:

Nursing care facilities	$9.11
Residential mental retardation, mental health and substance abuse facilities	8.97
Home health care services	8.57
Community care facilities for the elderly	8.57
Individual and family services	8.47

Home health aides receive slight pay increases with experience and added responsibility. Usually, they are paid only for the time worked in the home, not for travel time between jobs. Most employers hire only on-call hourly workers and provide no benefits.

Median hourly earnings of psychiatric aides were $11.19 in May 2004. The middle 50 percent earned between $9.09 and $14.09 an hour. The lowest 10 percent earned less than $7.63 and the highest 10 percent earned more than $16.74 an hour. Median hourly earnings in the industries employing the largest numbers of psychiatric aides in May 2004 were as follows:

General medical and surgical hospitals	$11.31
Psychiatric and substance abuse hospitals	11.06
Residential mental retardation, mental health and substance abuse facilities	9.37

Surgical Technologists

Significant Points: Employment is expected to grow much faster than the average for all occupations through the year 2014.

Job opportunities are expected to be good.

Training programmes last 9 to 24 months and lead to a certificate, diploma, or associate degree.

Hospitals will continue to be the primary employer, although much faster employment growth is expected in offices of physicians and in outpatient care centres, including ambulatory surgical centres.

Nature of the Work: Surgical technologists, also called scrubs and surgical or operating room technicians, assist in surgical operations under the supervision of surgeons, registered nurses, or other surgical personnel. Surgical technologists are members of operating room teams, which most commonly include surgeons, anesthesiologists and circulating nurses. Before an operation, surgical technologists help prepare the operating room by setting up surgical instruments and equipment, sterile drapes and sterile solutions.

They assemble both sterile and nonsterile equipment, as well as adjust and check it to ensure it is working properly. Technologists also get patients ready for surgery by washing, shaving and disinfecting incision sites. They transport patients to the operating room, help position them on the operating table and cover them with sterile surgical "drapes." Technologists also observe patients' vital signs, check charts and assist the surgical team with putting on sterile gowns and gloves.

During surgery, technologists pass instruments and other sterile supplies to surgeons and surgeon assistants. They may hold retractors, cut sutures and help count sponges, needles, supplies and instruments. Surgical technologists help prepare, care for and dispose of specimens taken for laboratory analysis and help apply dressings. Some operate sterilizers, lights, or suction machines and help operate diagnostic equipment.

After an operation, surgical technologists may help transfer patients to the recovery room and clean and restock the operating room.

Working Conditions: Surgical technologists work in clean, well-lighted, cool environments. They must stand for long periods and remain alert during operations. At times they may be exposed to communicable diseases and unpleasant sights, odours and materials.

Most surgical technologists work a regular 40-hour week, although they may be on call or work nights, weekends and holidays on a rotating basis.

Training, Other Qualifications and Advancement: Surgical technologists receive their training in formal programmes offered by community and junior colleges, vocational schools, universities, hospitals and the military. In 2005, the Commission on Accreditation of Allied Health Education Programmes (CAAHEP) recognized more than 400 accredited programmes. Programmes last from 9 to 24 months and lead to a certificate, diploma, or associate degree. High school graduation normally is required for admission. Recommended high school courses include health, biology, chemistry and mathematics.

Programmes provide classroom education and supervised clinical experience. Students take courses in anatomy, physiology, microbiology, pharmacology, professional ethics and medical terminology. Other studies cover the care and safety of patients during surgery, sterile techniques and surgical procedures. Students also learn to sterilize instruments; prevent and control infection; and handle special drugs, solutions, supplies and equipment.

Most employers prefer to hire certified technologists. Technologists may obtain voluntary professional certification from the Liaison Council on Certification for the Surgical Technologist by graduating from a CAAHEP-accredited programme and passing a national certification examination. They may then use the Certified Surgical Technologist (CST) designation. Continuing education or re-examination is required to maintain certification, which must be renewed every 4 years.

Certification also may be obtained from the National Centre for Competency Testing. To qualify to take the exam, candidates follow one of three paths: complete an accredited training programme; undergo a 2-year hospital on-the-job training programme; or acquire seven years of experience working in the field. After passing the exam, individuals may use the designation Tech in Surgery-Certified, TS-C (NCCT). This certification may be renewed every 5 years through either continuing education or re-examination.

Surgical technologists need manual dexterity to handle instruments quickly. They also must be conscientious, orderly and emotionally stable to handle the demands of the operating room environment. Technologists must respond quickly and must be familiar with operating procedures in order to have instruments ready for surgeons without having to be told. They are expected to keep abreast of new developments in the field.

Technologists advance by specializing in a particular area of surgery, such as neurosurgery or open heart surgery. They also may work as circulating technologists. A circulating technologist is the "unsterile" member of the surgical team who prepares patients; helps with anesthesia; obtains and opens packages for the "sterile" persons to remove the sterile contents during the procedure; interviews the patient before surgery; keeps a written account of the surgical procedure; and answers the surgeon's questions about the patient during the surgery. With additional training, some technologists advance to first assistants, who help with retracting, sponging, suturing, cauterizing bleeders and closing and treating wounds. Some surgical technologists manage central supply departments in hospitals, or take positions with insurance companies, sterile supply services and operating equipment firms.

Employment: Surgical technologists held about 84,000 jobs in 2004. About 7 out of 10 jobs for surgical technologists were in hospitals, mainly in operating and delivery rooms. Other jobs were in offices of physicians or dentists who perform outpatient surgery and in outpatient care centres, including ambulatory surgical centres. A few, known as private scrubs, are employed directly by surgeons who have special surgical teams, like those for liver transplants.

Job Outlook: Employment of surgical technologists is expected to grow much faster than average for all occupations through the year 2014 as the volume of surgery increases. Job opportunities are expected to be good. The number of surgical procedures is expected to rise as the population grows and ages. The number of older people, including the baby boom generation, who generally require more surgical procedures, will account for a larger portion of the general population. Technological advances, such as fiber optics and laser technology, will permit an increasing number of new surgical procedures to be performed and also will allow surgical technologists to assist with a greater number of procedures.

Hospitals will continue to be the primary employer of surgical technologists, although much faster employment growth is expected in offices of physicians and in outpatient care centres, including ambulatory surgical centres.

Earnings: Median annual earnings of surgical technologists were $34,010 in May 2004. The middle 50 percent earned between $28,560 and $40,750. The lowest 10 percent earned less than $23,940 and the highest 10 percent earned more than $45,990. Median hourly earnings in the industries employing the largest numbers of surgical technologists in May 2004 were:

Offices of dentists	$37,510
Offices of physicians	36,570
General medical and surgical hospitals	33,130

Radiologic Technologists and Technicians

Significant Points: Job opportunities are expected to be favourable; some employers report difficulty hiring sufficient numbers of radiologic technologists and technicians.

Formal training programmes in radiography range in length from 1 to 4 years and lead to a certificate, an associate degree, or a bachelor's degree.

Although hospitals will remain the primary employer, a greater number of new jobs will be found in physicians' offices and diagnostic imaging centres.

Nature of the Work: Radiologic technologists and technicians take x rays and administer non-radioactive materials into patients' bloodstreams for diagnostic purposes. Some specialize in diagnostic imaging technologies, such as computerized tomography (CT) and magnetic resonance imaging (MRI).

In addition to radiologic technologists and technicians, others who conduct diagnostic imaging procedures include cardiovascular technologists and technicians, diagnostic medical sonographers and nuclear medicine technologists. (Each is discussed elsewhere in the *Handbook.)*

Radiologic technologists and technicians, also referred to as *radiographers*, produce x-ray films (radiographs) of parts of the human body for use in diagnosing medical problems. They prepare patients for radiologic examinations by explaining the procedure, removing articles such as jewellery, through which x rays cannot pass and positioning patients so that the parts of the body can be appropriately radiographed.

To prevent unnecessary exposure to radiation, these workers surround the exposed area with radiation protection devices, such as lead shields, or limit the size of the x-ray beam. Radiographers position radiographic equipment at the correct angle and height over the appropriate area of a patient's body. Using instruments similar to a measuring tape, they may measure the thickness of the section to be radiographed and set controls on the x-ray machine to produce radiographs of the appropriate density, detail and contrast. They place the x-ray film under the part of the patient's body to be examined and make the exposure. They then remove the film and develop it.

Experienced radiographers may perform more complex imaging procedures. For fluoroscopies, radiographers prepare a solution of contrast medium for the patient to drink, allowing the radiologist (a physician who interprets radiographs) to see soft tissues in the body. Some radiographers, called *CT technologists,* operate CT scanners to produce cross-sectional images of patients. Radiographers who operate machines that use strong magnets and radio waves, rather than radiation, to create an image are called *MRI technologists*.

Radiologic technologists and technicians must follow physicians' orders precisely and conform to regulations concerning the use of radiation to protect themselves, their patients and their coworkers from unnecessary exposure.

In addition to preparing patients and operating equipment, radiologic technologists and technicians keep patient records and adjust and maintain equipment. They also may prepare work schedules, evaluate purchases of equipment, or manage a radiology department.

Working Conditions: Most full-time radiologic technologists and technicians work about 40 hours a week. They may, however, have evening, weekend, or on-call hours. Opportunities for part-time and shift work also are available.

Physical stamina is important, because technologists and technicians are on their feet for long periods and may lift or turn disabled patients. Technologists and technicians work at diagnostic machines, but also may perform some procedures at patients' bedsides. Some travel to patients in large vans equipped with sophisticated diagnostic equipment.

Although radiation hazards exist in this occupation, they are minimized by the use of lead aprons, gloves and other shielding devices, as well as by instruments monitoring exposure to radiation. Technologists and technicians wear badges measuring radiation levels in the radiation area and detailed records are kept on their cumulative lifetime dose.

Training, Other Qualifications and Advancement: Preparation for this profession is offered in hospitals, colleges and universities, vocational-technical institutes and the U.S. Armed Forces. Hospitals, which employ most radiologic technologists and technicians, prefer to hire those with formal training.

Formal training programmes in radiography range in length from 1 to 4 years and lead to a certificate, an associate degree, or a bachelor's degree. Two-year associate degree programmes are most prevalent.

Some 1-year certificate programmes are available for experienced radiographers or individuals from other health occupations, such as medical technologists and registered nurses, who want to change fields or specialize in CT or MRI. A bachelor's or master's degree in one of the radiologic technologies is desirable for supervisory, administrative, or teaching positions.

The Joint Review Committee on Education in Radiologic Technology accredits most formal training programmes for the field. The committee accredited 606 radiography programmes in 2005. Radiography programmes require, at a minimum, a high school diploma or the equivalent. High school courses in mathematics, physics, chemistry and biology are helpful. The programmes provide both classroom and clinical instruction in anatomy and physiology, patient care procedures, radiation physics, radiation protection, principles of imaging, medical terminology, positioning of patients, medical ethics, radiobiology and pathology.

Federal legislation protects the public from the hazards of unnecessary exposure to medical and dental radiation by ensuring that operators of radiologic equipment are properly trained. Under this legislation, the Federal Government sets voluntary standards that the States may use for accrediting training programmes and certifying individuals who engage in medical or dental radiography.

In 2005, 38 States certified radiologic technologists and technicians. Certification, which is voluntary, is offered by the American Registry of Radiologic Technologists. To be eligible for certification, technologists generally must graduate from an accredited programme and pass an examination. Many employers prefer to hire certified radiographers. To be recertified, radiographers must complete 24 hours of continuing education every two years.

Radiologic technologists and technicians should be sensitive to patients' physical and psychological needs. They must pay attention to detail, follow instructions and work as part of a team. In addition, operating complicated equipment requires mechanical ability and manual dexterity.

With experience and additional training, staff technologists may become specialists, performing CT scanning, angiography and magnetic resonance imaging. Experienced technologists also may be promoted to supervisor, chief radiologic technologist and, ultimately, department administrator or director. Depending on the institution, courses or a master's degree in business or health administration may be necessary for the director's position. Some technologists progress by leaving the occupation to become instructors or directors in radiologic technology programmes; others take jobs as sales representatives or instructors with equipment manufacturers.

Employment: Radiologic technologists and technicians held about 182,000 jobs in 2004. More than half of all jobs were in hospitals. Most of the rest were in offices of physicians; medical and diagnostic laboratories, including diagnostic imaging centres; and outpatient care centres.

Job Outlook: Job opportunities are expected to be favourable. Some employers report difficulty hiring sufficient numbers of radiologic technologists and technicians. Imbalances between the demand for and supply of, radiologic technologists and technicians should spur efforts to attract and retain qualified workers, such as improved compensation and working conditions. Radiologic technologists who also are experienced in more complex diagnostic imaging procedures, such as CT and MRI, will have better employment opportunities, brought about as employers seek to control costs by using multi-skilled employees.

Employment of radiologic technologists and technicians is expected to grow faster than the average for all occupations through 2014, as the population grows and ages, increasing the demand for diagnostic imaging. Although healthcare providers are enthusiastic about the clinical benefits of new technologies, the extent to which they are adopted depends largely on cost and reimbursement considerations. For example, digital imaging technology can improve the quality of the images and the efficiency of the procedure, but remains expensive. Some promising new technologies may not come into widespread use because they are too expensive and third-party payers may not be willing to pay for their use.

Hospitals will remain the principal employer of radiologic technologists and technicians. However, a greater number of new jobs will be found in offices of physicians and diagnostic imaging centres. Health facilities such as these are expected to grow rapidly through 2014, due to the strong shift toward outpatient care, encouraged by third-party payers and made possible by technological advances that permit more procedures to be performed outside the hospital. Some job openings also will arise from the need to replace technologists and technicians who leave the occupation.

Earnings: Median annual earnings of radiologic technologists and technicians were $43,350 in May 2004. The middle 50 percent earned between $36,170 and $52,430. The lowest 10 percent earned less than $30,020 and the highest 10 percent earned more than $60,210. Median annual earnings in the industries employing the largest numbers of radiologic technologists and technicians in May 2004 were:

Medical and diagnostic laboratories	$46,620
General medical and surgical hospitals	43,960
Offices of physicians	40,290

Occupational Health and Safety Specialists and Technicians

Significant Points: About 2 out of 5 specialists worked in Federal, State and local government agencies that enforce rules on safety, health and the environment.

Many employers, including the Federal Government, require a bachelor's degree in occupational health, safety, or a related field for some specialist positions.

Projected average employment growth reflects a balance of continuing public demand for a safe and healthy work environment against the desire for smaller government and fewer regulations.

Nature of the Work: Occupational health and safety specialists and technicians, also known as *safety and health practitioners* or *occupational health and safety inspectors*, help prevent harm to workers, property, the environment and the general public. They promote occupational health and safety within organizations in many ways, such as by advising management on how to increase worker productivity through raising morale and reducing absenteeism, turnover and equipment downtime while securing savings on insurance premiums, workers' compensation benefits and litigation expenses.

Occupational health and safety specialists analyze work environments and design programmes to control, eliminate and prevent disease or injury caused by chemical, physical, radiological and biological agents or ergonomic factors that involve the impact of equipment design on a worker's comfort or fatigue. They may conduct inspections and inform the management of a business which areas may not be in compliance with State and Federal laws or employer policies, in order to gain their support for addressing these areas. They advise management on the cost and effectiveness of safety and health programmes.

Occupational health and safety technicians collect data on work environments for analysis by occupational health and safety specialists. Usually working under the supervision of specialists, they help implement and evaluate programmes designed to limit risks to workers.

The specific responsibilities of occupational health and safety specialists and technicians vary by industry, workplace and types of hazards affecting employees. In most settings, they initially focus on identifying hazardous conditions and practices. Sometimes they develop methods to predict hazards from experience, historical data, workplace analysis and other information sources.

Then they identify potential hazards in systems, equipment, products, facilities, or processes planned for use in the future. For example, they might uncover patterns in injury data that implicate a specific cause such as system failure, human error, incomplete or faulty decision making, or a weakness in existing policies or practices.

After reviewing the causes or effects of hazards, they evaluate the probability and severity of accidents or exposures to hazardous materials that may result. Then they identify where controls need to be implemented to reduce or eliminate hazards and advise if a new programme or practice is required. As necessary, they conduct training sessions for management, supervisors and workers on health and safety practices and regulations to promote an understanding of a new or existing process. After implementation, they may monitor and evaluate the program's progress, making additional suggestions when needed.

To ensure the machinery and equipment meet appropriate safety regulations, occupational health and safety specialists and technicians may examine and test machinery and equipment, such as lifting devices, machine guards, or scaffolding. They may check that personal protective equipment, such as masks, respirators, protective eyewear, or hardhats, is being used in workplaces according to regulations.

]They also check that hazardous materials are stored correctly. They test and identify work areas for potential accident and health hazards, such as toxic vapors, mold, mildew and explosive gas-air mixtures and help implement appropriate control measures, such as adjustments to ventilation systems. Their survey of the workplace might involve talking with workers and observing their work, as well as inspecting elements in their work environment, such as lighting, tools and equipment.

To measure and control hazardous substances, such as the noise or radiation levels, occupational health and safety specialists and technicians prepare and calibrate scientific equipment. They must properly collect and handle samples of dust, gaspes, vapors and other potentially toxic materials to ensure personal safety and accurate test results.

If an injury or illness occurs, occupational health and safety specialists and technicians help investigate unsafe working conditions, study possible causes and recommend remedial action. Some occupational health and safety specialists and technicians assist with the rehabilitation of workers after accidents and injuries and make sure they return to work successfully.

Frequent communication with management may be necessary to report on the status of occupational health and safety programmes. Consultation with engineers or physicians also may be required.

Occupational health and safety specialists and technicians prepare reports including accident reports, Occupational Safety and Health Administration record-keeping forms, observations, analysis of contaminants and recommendations for control and correction of hazards. They may prepare documents to be used in legal proceedings and give testimony in court proceedings. Those who develop expertise in certain areas may develop occupational health and safety systems, including policies, procedures and manuals.

Specialists and technicians that concentrate in particular areas include environmental protection officers, ergonomists, health physicists, industrial hygienists and mine examiners. Environmental protection officers evaluate and coordinate programmes that impact the environment, such as the storage and handling of hazardous waste or monitoring the cleanup of contaminated soil or water. Ergonomists help ensure that the work environment allows employees to maximize their comfort, safety and productivity. Health physicists help protect people and the environment from hazardous radiation exposure by monitoring the manufacture, handling and disposal of radioactive material. Industrial hygienists examine the workplace for health hazards, such as worker exposure to lead, asbestos, pesticides, or communicable diseases. Mine examiners are technicians who inspect mines for proper air flow and health hazards such as the buildup of methane or other noxious gases.

Working Conditions: Occupational health and safety specialists and technicians work with many different people in a variety of environments. Their jobs often involve considerable fieldwork and some travel frequently. Many occupational health and safety specialists and technicians work long and often irregular hours.

Occupational health and safety specialists and technicians may be exposed to many of the same physically strenuous conditions and hazards as industrial employees and the work may be performed in unpleasant, stressful and dangerous working conditions. They may find themselves in an adversarial role if the management of an organization disagrees with the recommendations for ensuring a safe working environment.

Training, Other Qualifications and Advancement: All occupational health and safety specialists and technicians are trained in the applicable laws or inspection procedures through some combination of classroom and on-the-job training. Awards and degrees in programmes related to occupational safety and health include 1-year certificates, associate degrees, bachelor's degrees and graduate degrees.

The Accreditation Board for Engineering and Technology (ABET) accredits health physics, industrial hygiene and safety programmes, in addition to engineering programmes. Many employers, including the Federal Government, require a bachelor's degree in occupational health, safety, or a related field, such as engineering, biology, or chemistry, for some specialist positions. Many industrial hygiene programmes result in a master's degree. Experience as an occupational health and safety professional is also a prerequisite for many positions. Advancement to senior specialist positions is likely to require an advanced degree and substantial experience in several areas of practice.

In general, people who want to enter this occupation should be responsible and like detailed work. Occupational health and safety specialists and technicians should be able to communicate well. Recommended high school courses include English, mathematics, chemistry, biology and physics.

Certification is available through the Board of Certified Safety Professionals (BCSP) and the American Board of Industrial .Hygiene (ABIH). The BCSP offers the Certified Safety Professional (CSP) credential, while the ABIH offers the Certified Industrial Hygienist (CIH) and Certified Associate Industrial Hygienist (CAIH) credentials. Also, the Council on Certification of Health, Environmental and Safety Technologists, a joint effort between the BCSP and ABIH, awards the Occupational Health and Safety Technologist (OHST) and Construction Health and Safety Technician (CHST) credentials. Requirements for the OHST and CHST credentials are less stringent than those for the CSP, CIH, or CAIH credentials. Once education and experience requirements have been met, certification may be obtained through an examination. Continuing education is required for recertification. Although voluntary, many employers encourage certification.

Federal Government occupational health and safety specialists and technicians whose job performance is satisfactory advance through their career ladder to a specified full-performance level. For positions above this level, usually supervisory positions, advancement is competitive and based on agency needs and individual merit. Advancement opportunities in State and local governments and the private sector are often similar to those in the Federal Government.

Research or related teaching positions at the college level require advanced education.

Employment: Occupational health and safety specialists held about 40,000 jobs in 2004. While the majority of jobs were spread throughout the private sector, about 2 out of 5 specialists worked for government agencies. Local governments employed 19 percent, State governments employed 18 percent and the Federal Government employed 4 percent. Other occupational health and safety specialists were employed in manufacturing firms; private general medical and surgical hospitals; management, scientific and technical consulting services; management of companies and enterprises; support activities for mining; research and development in the physical, engineering and life sciences; private colleges, universities and professional schools; and electric power generation, transmission and distribution. Some were self-employed.

Occupational health and safety technicians held about 12,000 jobs in 2004. Nearly 3 out of 10 technicians worked in government agencies. Local governments employed 13 percent, State governments employed 7 percent and the Federal Government employed 9 percent. Other occupational health and safety technicians were employed in manufacturing firms; private general medical and surgical hospitals; private colleges, universities and professional schools; employment services; management, scientific and technical consulting services; testing laboratories for architectural, engineering and related services; research and development in the physical, engineering and life sciences; and electric power generation, transmission and distribution.

Within the Federal Government, most jobs are as Occupational Safety and Health Administration (OSHA) inspectors, who enforce U.S. Department of Labour regulations that ensure adequate safety principles, practices and techniques are applied in workplaces. Employers may be fined for violation of OSHA standards.

Within the U.S. Department of Health and Human Services, occupational health and safety specialists working for the National Institute of Occupational Safety and Health (NIOSH) provide private companies with an avenue to evaluate the health and safety of their employees without the risk of being fined. Most large government agencies also employ occupational health and safety specialists and technicians who work to protect agency employees.

Most private companies either employ their own occupational health and safety personnel or contract with occupational health and safety professionals to ensure the safety of their workers and compliance with Federal, State and local government agencies that enforce rules on safety, health and the environment.

Job Outlook: Employment of occupational health and safety specialists and technicians is expected to grow about as fast as average for all occupations through 2014, reflecting a balance of continuing public demand for a safe and healthy work environment against the desire for smaller government and fewer regulations. Since the September 11, 2001 attacks, emergency preparedness has become a greater focus for the public and private sectors and for occupational health and safety specialists and technicians.

Additional job openings will arise from the need to replace those who transfer to other occupations, retire, or leave for other reasons. In private industry, employment growth will reflect industry growth and the continuing self-enforcement of government and company regulations and policies.

Employment of occupational health and safety specialists and technicians in the private sector is somewhat affected by general economic fluctuations. Federal, State and local governments, which employ about 2 out of 5 of all specialists and technicians, provide considerable job security; workers are less likely to be affected by changes in the economy.

Earnings: Median annual earnings of occupational health and safety specialists were $51,570 in May 2004. The middle 50 percent earned between $39,580 and $65,370. The lowest 10 percent earned less than $30,590 and the highest 10 percent earned more than $79,530. Median annual earnings of occupational health and safety specialists in May 2004 were $48,710 in local government and $44,400 in State government.

Median annual earnings of occupational health and safety technicians were $42,130 in May 2004. The middle 50 percent earned between $29,900 and $56,640. The lowest 10 percent earned less than $22,860 and the highest 10 percent earned more than $70,460. Most occupational health and safety specialists and technicians work in large private firms or for Federal, State and local governments, most of which generally offer more generous benefits than smaller firms.

Medical and Health Services Managers

Significant Points: Rapid employment growth is projected; job opportunities will be especially good in offices of health practitioners, general medical and surgical hospitals, home health care services and outpatient care centres.

Applicants with work experience in health care and strong business and management skills likely will have the best opportunities.

Earnings are high, but long work hours are common.

A master's degree is the standard credential for most positions, although a bachelor's degree is adequate for some entry-level positions in smaller facilities and in health information management.

Nature of the Work: Health care is a business and, like every other business, it needs good management to keep it running smoothly. Medical and health services managers, also referred to as *health care executives* or *health care administrators*, plan, direct, coordinate and supervise the delivery of health care. Medical and health services managers include specialists and generalists. Specialists are in charge of specific clinical departments or services, while generalists manage or help manage an entire facility or system.

The structure and financing of health care are changing rapidly. Future medical and health services managers must be prepared to deal with evolving integrated health care delivery systems, technological innovations, an increasingly complex regulatory environment, restructuring of work and an increased focus on preventive care.

They will be called on to improve efficiency in health care facilities and the quality of the health care provided. Increasingly, medical and health services managers will work in organizations in which they must optimize efficiency of a variety of related services—for example, those ranging from inpatient care to outpatient followup care.

Large facilities usually have several assistant administrators to aid the top administrator and to handle daily decisions. Assistant administrators may direct activities in clinical areas such as nursing, surgery, therapy, medical records, or health information. (Managers in non-health areas, such as administrative services, computer and information systems, finance and human resources, are not included in this statement.

In smaller facilities, top administrators handle more of the details of daily operations. For example, many nursing home administrators manage personnel, finances, facility operations and admissions and also have a larger role in resident care.

Clinical managers have training or experience in a specific clinical area and, accordingly, have more specific responsibilities than do generalists. For example, directors of physical therapy are experienced physical therapists and most health information and medical record administrators have a bachelor's degree in health information or medical record administration. Clinical managers establish and implement policies, objectives and procedures for their departments; evaluate personnel and work; develop reports and budgets; and coordinate activities with other managers.

Health information managers are responsible for the maintenance and security of all patient records. Recent regulations enacted by the Federal Government require that all health care providers maintain electronic patient records and that these records be secure. As a result, health information managers must keep up with current computer and software technology and with legislative requirements and developments. In addition, as patient data become more frequently used for quality management and in medical research, health information managers ensure that databases are complete, accurate and available only to authorized personnel.

In group medical practices, managers work closely with physicians. Whereas an office manager might handle business affairs in small medical groups, leaving policy decisions to the physicians themselves, larger groups usually employ a full-time administrator to help formulate business strategies and coordinate day-to-day business.

A small group of 10 to 15 physicians might employ 1 administrator to oversee personnel matters, billing and collection, budgeting, planning, equipment outlays and patient flow. A large practice of 40 to 50 physicians might have a chief administrator and several assistants, each responsible for different areas.

Medical and health services managers in managed care settings perform functions similar to those of their counterparts in large group practices, except that they could have larger staffs to manage. In addition, they might do more community outreach and preventive care than do managers of a group practice. Some medical and health services managers oversee the activities of a number of facilities in health systems. Such systems might contain both inpatient and outpatient facilities and offer a wide range of patient services.

Working Conditions: Most medical and health services managers work long hours. Facilities such as nursing care facilities and hospitals operate around the clock and administrators and managers may be called at all hours to deal with problems. They also may travel to attend meetings or inspect satellite facilities.

Some managers work in comfortable, private offices; others share space with other managers or staff. They may spend considerable time walking, to consult with coworkers.

Training, Other Qualifications and Advancement: Medical and health services managers must be familiar with management principles and practices. A master's degree in health services administration, long-term care administration, health sciences, public health, public administration, or business administration is the standard credential for most generalist positions in this field. However, a bachelor's degree is adequate for some entry-level positions in smaller facilities, at the departmental level within health care organizations and in health information management. Physicians' offices and some other facilities may substitute on-the-job experience for formal education.

Bachelor's, master's and doctoral degree programmes in health administration are offered by colleges; universities; and schools of public health, medicine, allied health, public administration and business administration. In 2005, 70 schools had accredited programmes leading to the master's degree in health services administration, according to the Commission on Accreditation of Healthcare Management Education.

For persons seeking to become heads of clinical departments, a degree in the appropriate field and work experience may be sufficient early in their career. However, a master's degree in health services administration or a related field might be required to advance. For example, nursing service administrators usually are chosen from among supervisory registered nurses with administrative abilities and graduate degrees in nursing or health services administration.

Health information managers require a bachelor's degree from an accredited programme and a Registered Health Information Administrator (RHIA) certification from the

American Health Information Management Association. In 2005, there were 45 accredited bachelor's programmes in health information management according to the Commission on Accreditation for Health Informatics and Information Management Education.

Some graduate programmes seek students with undergraduate degrees in business or health administration; however, many graduate programmes prefer students with a liberal arts or health profession background. Candidates with previous work experience in health care also may have an advantage. Competition for entry into these programmes is keen and applicants need above-average grades to gain admission. Graduate programmes usually last between 2 and 3 years.

They may include up to 1 year of supervised administrative experience and coursework in areas such as hospital organization and management, marketing, accounting and budgeting, human resources administration, strategic planning, law and ethics, biostatistics or epidemiology, health economics and health information systems. Some programmes allow students to specialize in one type of facility—hospitals, nursing care facilities, mental health facilities, or medical groups. Other programmes encourage a generalist approach to health administration education.

New graduates with master's degrees in health services administration may start as department managers or as staff. The level of the starting position varies with the experience of the applicant and the size of the organization. Hospitals and other health facilities offer postgraduate residencies and fellowships, which usually are staff positions. Graduates from master's degree programmes also take jobs in large medical group practices, clinics, mental health facilities, nursing care corporations and consulting firms.

Graduates with bachelor's degrees in health administration usually begin as administrative assistants or assistant department heads in larger hospitals. They also may begin as department heads or assistant administrators in small hospitals or nursing care facilities.

All States and the District of Columbia require nursing care facility administrators to have a bachelor's degree, pass a licensing examination, complete a State-approved training programme and pursue continuing education. Some States also require licenses for administrators in assisted living facilities. A license is not required in other areas of medical and health services management.

Medical and health services managers often are responsible for millions of dollars' worth of facilities and equipment and hundreds of employees. To make effective decisions, they need to be open to different opinions and good at analyzing contradictory information. They must understand finance and information systems and be able to interpret data. Motivating others to implement their decisions requires strong leadership abilities. Tact, diplomacy, flexibility and communication skills are essential because medical and health services managers spend most of their time interacting with others.

Medical and health services managers advance by moving into more responsible and higher paying positions, such as assistant or associate administrator, department head, or CEO, or by moving to larger facilities. Some experienced managers also may become consultants or professors of health care management.

Employment: Medical and health services managers held about 248,000 jobs in 2004. About 30 percent worked in private hospitals and another 16 percent worked in offices of physicians or in nursing care facilities. The remainder worked mostly in home health care services, Federal Government health care facilities, ambulatory facilities run by State and local governments, outpatient care centres, insurance carriers and community care facilities for the elderly.

Job Outlook: Employment of medical and health services managers is expected to grow faster than average for all occupations through 2014, as the health care industry continues to expand and diversify. Job opportunities will be especially good in offices of health practitioners, general medical and surgical hospitals, home health care services and outpatient care centres. Applicants with work experience in the health care field and strong business and management skills should have the best opportunities. Competition for jobs at the highest management levels will be keen because of the high pay and prestige.

Managers in all settings will be needed to improve quality and efficiency of health care while controlling costs, as insurance companies and Medicare demand higher levels of accountability. Managers also will be needed to computerize patient records and to ensure their security as required by law. Additional demand for managers will stem from the need to recruit workers and increase employee retention, to comply with changing regulations, to implement new technology and to help improve the health of their communities by emphasizing preventive care.

Hospitals will continue to employ the most medical and health services managers over the 2004-14 projection period. However, the number of new jobs created is expected to increase at a slower rate in hospitals than in many other industries because of the growing utilization of clinics and other outpatient care sites. Despite relatively slow employment growth, a large number of new jobs will be created because of the industry's large size. Medical and health services managers with experience in large facilities will enjoy the best job opportunities, as hospitals become larger and more complex.

Employment will grow fastest in practitioners' offices and in home health care agencies. Many services previously provided in hospitals will continue to shift to these sectors, especially as medical technologies improve. Demand in medical group practice management will grow as medical group practices become larger and more complex. Managers with specialized experience in a particular field, such as reimbursement, should have good opportunities.

Medical and health services managers also will be employed by health care management companies that provide management services to hospitals and other organizations, as well as to specific departments such as emergency, information management systems, managed care contract negotiations and physician recruiting.

Earnings: Median annual earnings of medical and health services managers were $67,430 in May 2004. The middle 50 percent earned between $52,530 and $88,210. The lowest 10 percent earned less than $41,450 and the highest 10 percent earned more than $117,990. Median annual earnings in the industries employing the largest numbers of medical and health services managers in May 2004 were as follows:

Federal Government	$87,200
General medical and surgical hospitals	71,280
Offices of physicians	61,320
Nursing care facilities	60,940
Home health care services	60,320

Earnings of medical and health services managers vary by type and size of the facility, as well as by level of responsibility. For example, the Medical Group Management Association reported that, in 2004, median salaries for administrators were $72,875 in practices with 6 or fewer physicians, $95,766 in practices with 7 to 25 physicians and $132,955 in practices with 26 or more physicians.

According to a survey by *Modern Healthcare* magazine, median annual compensation in 2004 for hospital administrators of selected clinical departments was $76,800 in respiratory care, $81,100 in physical therapy, $87,700 in home health care, $88,800 in laboratory services, $90,200 in long-term care, $93,500 in medical imaging/diagnostic radiology, $94,400 in rehabilitation services, $95,200 in cancer treatment facilities, $96,200 in cardiology, $102,800 in nursing services and $113,200 in pharmacies. Salaries also varied according to size of facility and geographic region.

According to a survey by the Professional Association of Health Care Office Management, total 2004 median compensation for office managers in speciality physicians' practices was $72,047 in gastroenterology, $66,946 in dermatology, $66,207 in cardiology, $64,543 in ophthalmology, $63,801 in obstetrics and gynecology, $62,545 in orthopedics, $58,595 in pediatrics, $52,211 in internal medicine, $50,924 in psychiatry and $50,049 in family practice.

Emergency Medical Technicians and Paramedics

Significant Points: Because emergency services function 24 hours a day, emergency medical technicians and paramedics have irregular working hours.

Emergency medical technicians and paramedics need formal training and certification, but requirements vary by State.

Employment is projected to grow much faster than average as paid emergency medical technician positions replace unpaid volunteers. Competition will be greater for jobs in local fire, police and rescue squad departments than in private ambulance services; opportunities will be best for those who have advanced certification.

Nature of the Work: People's lives often depend on the quick reaction and competent care of emergency medical technicians (EMTs) and paramedics—EMTs with additional advanced training to perform more difficult prehospital medical procedures. Incidents as varied as automobile accidents, heart attacks, drownings, childbirth and gunshot wounds all require immediate medical attention. EMTs and paramedics provide this vital attention as they care for and transport the sick or injured to a medical facility.

In an emergency, EMTs and paramedics typically are dispatched to the scene by a 911 operator and often work with police and fire department personnel. (Police and detectives and firefighting occupations are discussed elsewhere in the *Handbook.*) Once they arrive, they determine the nature and extent of the patient's condition while trying to ascertain whether the patient has preexisting medical problems. Following strict rules and guidelines, they give appropriate emergency care and, when necessary, transport the patient. Some paramedics are trained to treat patients with minor injuries on the scene of an accident or at their home without transporting them to a medical facility. Emergency treatment for more complicated problems is carried out under the direction of medical doctors by radio preceding or during transport.

EMTs and paramedics may use special equipment, such as backboards, to immobilize patients before placing them on stretchers and securing them in the ambulance for transport to a medical facility. Usually, one EMT or paramedic drives while the other monitors the patient's vital signs and gives additional care as needed. Some EMTs work as part of the flight crew of helicopters that transport critically ill or injured patients to hospital trauma centres.

At the medical facility, EMTs and paramedics help transfer patients to the emergency department, report their observations and actions to emergency room staff and may provide additional emergency treatment. After each run, EMTs and paramedics replace used supplies and check equipment. If a transported patient had a contagious disease, EMTs and paramedics decontaminate the interior of the ambulance and report cases to the proper authorities.

Beyond these general duties, the specific responsibilities of EMTs and paramedics depend on their level of qualification and training. To determine this, the National Registry of Emergency Medical Technicians (NREMT) registers emergency medical service (EMS) providers at four levels: First Responder, EMT-Basic, EMT-Intermediate and EMT-Paramedic. Some States, however, do their own certification and use numeric ratings from 1 to 4 to distinguish levels of proficiency.

The lowest-level workers—First Responders—are trained to provide basic emergency medical care because they tend to be the first persons to arrive at the scene of an incident. Many firefighters, police officers and other emergency workers have this level of training. The EMT-Basic, also known as EMT-1, represents the first component of the emergency medical technician system. An EMT-1 is trained to care for patients at the scene of an accident and while transporting patients by ambulance to the hospital under medical direction. The EMT-1 has the emergency skills to assess a patient's condition and manage respiratory, cardiac and trauma emergencies.

The EMT-Intermediate (EMT-2 and EMT-3) has more advanced training that allows the administration of intravenous fluids, the use of manual defibrillators to give life-saving shocks to a stopped heart and the application of advanced airway techniques and equipment to assist patients experiencing respiratory emergencies. EMT-Paramedics (EMT-4) provide the most extensive prehospital care. In addition to carrying out the procedures already described, paramedics may administer drugs orally and intravenously, interpret electrocardiograms (EKGs), perform endotracheal intubations and use monitors and other complex equipment.

Working Conditions: EMTs and paramedics work both indoors and outdoors, in all types of weather. They are required to do considerable kneeling, bending and heavy lifting. These workers risk noise-induced hearing loss from sirens and back injuries from lifting patients. In addition, EMTs and paramedics may be exposed to diseases such as hepatitis-B and AIDS, as well as violence from drug overdose victims or mentally unstable patients. The work is not only physically strenuous, but can be stressful, sometimes involving life-or-death situations and suffering patients. Nonetheless, many people find the work exciting and challenging and enjoy the opportunity to help others.

EMTs and paramedics employed by fire departments work about 50 hours a week. Those employed by hospitals frequently work between 45 and 60 hours a week and those in private ambulance services, between 45 and 50 hours. Some of these workers, especially those in police and fire departments, are on call for extended periods. Because emergency services function 24 hours a day, EMTs and paramedics have irregular working hours.

Training, Other Qualifications and Advancement: Formal training and certification is needed to become an EMT or paramedic. A high school diploma is typically required to enter a formal training programme. Some programmes offer an associate degree along with the formal EMT training. All 50 States have a certification procedure. In most States and the District of Columbia, registration with the NREMT is required at some or all levels of certification. Other States administer their own certification examination or provide the option of taking the NREMT examination. To maintain certification, EMTs and paramedics must reregister, usually every 2 years. In order to reregister, an individual must be working as an EMT or paramedic and meet a continuing education requirement.

Training is offered at progressive levels: EMT-Basic, also known as EMT-1; EMT-Intermediate, or EMT-2 and EMT-3; and EMT-Paramedic, or EMT-4. EMT-Basic coursework typically emphasizes emergency skills, such as managing respiratory, trauma and cardiac emergencies and patient assessment. Formal courses are often combined with time in an emergency room or ambulance.

The programme also provides instruction and practice in dealing with bleeding, fractures, airway obstruction, cardiac arrest and emergency childbirth. Students learn how to use and maintain common emergency equipment, such as backboards, suction devices, splints, oxygen delivery systems and stretchers. Graduates of approved EMT basic training programmes who pass a written and practical examination administered by the State certifying agency or the NREMT earn the title "Registered EMT-Basic." The course also is a prerequisite for EMT-Intermediate and EMT-Paramedic training.

EMT-Intermediate training requirements vary from State to State. Applicants can opt to receive training in EMT-Shock Trauma, wherein the caregiver learns to start intravenous fluids and give certain medications, or in EMT-Cardiac, which includes learning heart rhythms and administering advanced medications. Training commonly includes 35 to 55 hours of additional instruction beyond EMT-Basic coursework and covers patient assessment as well as the use of advanced airway devices and intravenous fluids. Prerequisites for taking the EMT-Intermediate examination include registration as an EMT-Basic, required classroom work and a specified amount of clinical experience.

The most advanced level of training for this occupation is EMT-Paramedic. At this level, the caregiver receives additional training in body function and learns more advanced skills. The Technology programme usually lasts up to 2 years and results in an associate degree in applied science. Such education prepares the graduate to take the NREMT examination and become certified as an EMT-Paramedic. Extensive related coursework and clinical and field experience is required. Because of the longer training requirement, almost all EMT-Paramedics are in paid positions, rather than being volunteers. Refresher courses and continuing education are available for EMTs and paramedics at all levels.

EMTs and paramedics should be emotionally stable, have good dexterity, agility and physical coordination and be able to lift and carry heavy loads. They also need good eyesight (corrective lenses may be used) with accurate colour vision.

Advancement beyond the EMT-Paramedic level usually means leaving fieldwork. An EMT-Paramedic can become a supervisor, operations manager, administrative director, or executive director of emergency services. Some EMTs and paramedics become instructors, dispatchers, or physician assistants, while others move into sales or marketing of emergency medical equipment. A number of people become EMTs and paramedics to assess their interest in health care and then decide to return to school and become registered nurses, physicians, or other health workers.

Employment: EMTs and paramedics held about 192,000 jobs in 2004. Most career EMTs and paramedics work in metropolitan areas. Volunteer EMTs and paramedics are more common in small cities, towns and rural areas. These individuals volunteer for fire departments, emergency medical services (EMS), or hospitals and may respond to only a few calls for service per month or may answer the majority of calls, especially in smaller communities. EMTs and paramedics work closely with firefighters, who often are certified as EMTs as well and act as first responders. A large number of EMTs or paramedics belong to a union.

Full-time and part-time paid EMTs and paramedics were employed in a number of industries. About 4 out of 10 worked as employees of private ambulance services. About 3 out of 10 worked in local government for fire departments, public ambulance services and EMS. Another 2 out of 10 were found in hospitals, working full time within the medical facility or responding to calls in ambulances or helicopters to transport critically ill or injured patients. The remainder worked in various industries providing emergency services.

Job Outlook: Employment of emergency medical technicians and paramedics is expected to grow much faster than the average for all occupations through 2014, as full-time paid EMTs and paramedics replace unpaid volunteers. As population and urbanization increase and as a large segment of the population—aging baby boomers—becomes more likely to have medical emergencies, demand will increase for EMTs and paramedics.

There will still be demand for part-time, volunteer EMTs and paramedics in rural areas and smaller metropolitan areas. In addition to jobs arising from growth, openings will occur because of replacement needs; turnover is relatively high in this occupation because of the limited potential for advancement and the modest pay and benefits in private-sector jobs.

Job opportunities should be best in private ambulance services. Competition will be greater for jobs in local government, including fire, police and independent third-service rescue squad departments, in which salaries and benefits tend to be slightly better.

EMTs and paramedics who have advanced certifications, such as EMT-Intermediate and EMT-Paramedic, should enjoy the most favourable job prospects as clients and patients demand higher levels of care before arriving at the hospital.

Earnings: Earnings of EMTs and paramedics depend on the employment setting and geographic location as well as the individual's training and experience. Median annual earnings of EMTs and paramedics were $25,310 in May 2004. The middle 50 percent earned between $19,970 and $33,210. The lowest 10 percent earned less than $16,090 and the highest 10 percent earned more than $43,240. Median annual earnings in the industries employing the largest numbers of EMTs and paramedics in May 2004 were:

Local government	$27,710
General medical and surgical hospitals	26,590
Other ambulatory health care services	23,130

Those in emergency medical services who are part of fire or police departments receive the same benefits as firefighters or police officers. For example, many are covered by pension plans that provide retirement at half pay after 20 or 25 years of service or if the worker is disabled in the line of duty.

Physician Assistants

Significant Points: Physician assistant programmes usually last at least 2 years; admission requirements vary by programme, but many require at least 2 years of college and some health care experience.

All States require physician assistants to complete an accredited education programme and to pass a national exam in order to obtain a license.

Physician assistants rank among the fastest growing occupations, as physicians and health care institutions increasingly utilize physician assistants in order to contain costs.

Job opportunities should be good, particularly in rural and inner city clinics.

Nature of the Work: Physician assistants (PAs) practice medicine under the supervision of physicians and surgeons. They should not be confused with medical assistants, who perform routine clinical and clerical tasks. PAs are formally trained to provide diagnostic, therapeutic and preventive health care services, as delegated by a physician. Working as members of the health care team, they take medical histories, examine and treat patients, order and interpret laboratory tests and x-rays and make diagnoses.

They also treat minor injuries, by suturing, splinting and casting. PAs record progress notes, instruct and counsel patients and order or carry out therapy. In 48 States and the District of Columbia, physician assistants may prescribe medications. PAs also may have managerial duties. Some order medical supplies or equipment and supervise technicians and assistants.

Physician assistants work under the supervision of a physician. However, PAs may be the principal care providers in rural or inner city clinics, where a physician is present for only 1 or 2 days each week. In such cases, the PA confers with the supervising physician and other medical professionals as needed and as required by law. PAs also may make house calls or go to hospitals and nursing care facilities to check on patients, after which they report back to the physician.

The duties of physician assistants are determined by the supervising physician and by State law. Aspiring PAs should investigate the laws and regulations in the States in which they wish to practice.

Many PAs work in primary care specialities, such as general internal medicine, pediatrics and family medicine. Other speciality areas include general and thoracic surgery, emergency medicine, orthopedics and geriatrics. PAs specializing in surgery provide pre-operative and postoperative care and may work as first or second assistants during major surgery.

Working Conditions: Although PAs usually work in a comfortable, well-lighted environment, those in surgery often stand for long periods and others do considerable walking. Schedules vary according to the practice setting and often depend on the hours of the supervising physician. The workweek of hospital-based PAs may include weekends, nights, or early morning hospital rounds to visit patients. These workers also may be on call. PAs in clinics usually work a 40-hour week.

Training, Other Qualifications and Advancement: All States require that PAs complete an accredited, formal education programme and pass a National exam to obtain a license. PA programmes usually last at least 2 years and are full time. Most programmes are in schools of allied health, academic health centres, medical schools, or 4-year colleges; a few are in community colleges, the military, or hospitals. Many accredited PA programmes have clinical teaching affiliations with medical schools.

In 2005, more than 135 education programmes for physician assistants were accredited or provisionally accredited by the American Academy of Physician Assistants. More than 90 of these programmes offered the option of a master's degree and the rest offered either a bachelor's degree or an associate degree. Most applicants to PA educational programmes already have a bachelor's degree.

Admission requirements vary, but many programmes require 2 years of college and some work experience in the health care field. Students should take courses in biology, English, chemistry, mathematics, psychology and the social sciences. Many PAs have prior experience as registered nurses, while others come from varied backgrounds, including military corpsman/medics and allied health occupations such as respiratory therapists, physical therapists and emergency medical technicians and paramedics.

PA education includes classroom instruction in biochemistry, pathology, human anatomy, physiology, microbiology, clinical pharmacology, clinical medicine, geriatric and home health care, disease prevention and medical ethics. Students obtain supervised clinical training in several areas, including family medicine, internal medicine, surgery, prenatal care and gynecology, geriatrics, emergency medicine, psychiatry and pediatrics. Sometimes, PA students serve one or more of these "rotations" under the supervision of a physician who is seeking to hire a PA. The rotations often lead to permanent employment.

All States and the District of Columbia have legislation governing the qualifications or practice of physician assistants. All jurisdictions require physician assistants to pass the Physician Assistant National Certifying Examination, administered by the National Commission on Certification of Physician Assistants (NCCPA) and open only to graduates of accredited PA education programmes. Only those successfully completing the examination may use the credential "Physician Assistant-Certified." In order to remain certified, PAs must complete 100 hours of continuing medical education every 2 years. Every 6 years, they must pass a recertification examination or complete an alternative programme combining learning experiences and a take-home examination.

Some PAs pursue additional education in a speciality such as surgery, neonatology, or emergency medicine. PA postgraduate educational programmes are available in areas such as internal medicine, rural primary care, emergency medicine, surgery, pediatrics, neonatology and occupational medicine. Candidates must be graduates of an accredited programme and be certified by the NCCPA.

Physician assistants need leadership skills, self-confidence and emotional stability. They must be willing to continue studying throughout their career to keep up with medical advances. As they attain greater clinical knowledge and experience, PAs can advance to added responsibilities and higher earnings. However, by the very nature of the profession, clinically practicing PAs always are supervised by physicians.

Employment: Physician assistants held about 62,000 jobs in 2004. The number of jobs is greater than the number of practicing PAs because some hold two or more jobs. For example, some PAs work with a supervising physician, but also work in another practice, clinic, or hospital. According to the American Academy of Physician Assistants, about 15 percent of actively practicing PAs worked in more than one clinical job concurrently in 2004.

More than half of jobs for PAs were in the offices of physicians. About a quarter were in hospitals, public or private. The rest were mostly in outpatient care centres, including health maintenance organizations; the Federal Government; and public or private colleges, universities and professional schools. A few were self-employed.

Job Outlook: Employment of PAs is expected to grow much faster than average for all occupations through the year 2014, ranking among the fastest growing occupations, due to anticipated expansion of the health care industry and an emphasis on cost containment, resulting in increasing utilization of PAs by physicians and health care institutions.

Physicians and institutions are expected to employ more PAs to provide primary care and to assist with medical and surgical procedures because PAs are cost-effective and productive members of the health care team. Physician assistants can relieve physicians of routine duties and procedures. Telemedicine—using technology to facilitate interactive consultations between physicians and physician assistants—also will expand the use of physician assistants. Job opportunities for PAs should be good, particularly in rural and inner city clinics, because those settings have difficulty attracting physicians.

Besides the traditional office-based setting, PAs should find a growing number of jobs in institutional settings such as hospitals, academic medical centres, public clinics and prisons. Additional PAs may be needed to augment medical staffing in inpatient teaching hospital settings as the number of hours physician residents are permitted to work is reduced, encouraging hospitals to use PAs to supply some physician resident services. Opportunities will be best in States that allow PAs a wider scope of practice.

Earnings: Median annual earnings of physician assistants were $69,410 in May 2004. The middle 50 percent earned between $57,110 and $83,560. The lowest 10 percent earned less than $37,320 and the highest 10 percent earned more than $94,880. Median annual earnings of physician assistants in 2004 were $70,310 in general medical and surgical hospitals and $69,210 in offices of physicians.

According to the American Academy of Physician Assistants, median income for physician assistants in full-time clinical practice in 2004 was $74,264; median income for first-year graduates was $64,536. Income varies by speciality, practice setting, geographical location and years of experience. Employers often pay for their employees' liability insurance, registration fees with the Drug Enforcement Administration, State licensing fees and credentialing fees.

Cardiovascular Technologists and Technicians

Significant Points: About 3 out of 4 jobs were in hospitals.

The vast majority of cardiovascular technologists and technicians complete a 2-year junior or community college programme.

Employment will grow much faster than the average, but the number of job openings created will be low because the occupation is small.

Employment of most specialities will grow, but fewer EKG technicians will be needed.

Nature of the Work: Cardiovascular technologists and technicians assist physicians in diagnosing and treating cardiac (heart) and peripheral vascular (blood vessel) ailments. Cardiovascular technologists may specialize in any of three areas of practice: invasive cardiology, echocardiography and vascular technology. Cardiovascular technicians who specialize in electrocardiograms (EKGs), stress testing and Holter monitors are known as *cardiographic technicians*, or *EKG technicians*.

Cardiovascular technologists specializing in invasive procedures are called *cardiology technologists*. They assist physicians with cardiac catheterization procedures in which a small tube, or catheter, is threaded through a patient's artery from a spot on the patient's groin to the heart. The procedure can determine whether a blockage exists in the blood vessels that supply the heart muscle. The procedure also can help to diagnose other problems. Part of the procedure may involve balloon angioplasty, which can be used to treat blockages of blood vessels or heart valves without the need for heart surgery. Cardiology technologists assist physicians as they insert a catheter with a balloon on the end to the point of the obstruction.

Technologists prepare patients for cardiac catheterization and balloon angioplasty by first positioning them on an examining table and then shaving, cleaning and administering anesthesia to the top of their leg near the groin. During the procedures, they monitor patients' blood pressure and heart rate with EKG equipment and notify the physician if something appears to be wrong. Technologists also may prepare and monitor patients during open-heart surgery and during the insertion of pacemakers and stents that open up blockages in arteries to the heart and major blood vessels.

Cardiovascular technologists who specialize in echocardiography or vascular technology often run noninvasive tests using ultrasound instrumentation, such as Doppler ultrasound. Tests are called "noninvasive" if they do not require the insertion of probes or other instruments into the patient's body. The ultrasound instrumentation transmits high-frequency sound waves into areas of the patient's body and then processes reflected echoes of the sound waves to form an image. Technologists view the ultrasound image on a screen and may record the image on videotape or photograph it for interpretation and diagnosis by a physician. As the instrument scans the image, technologists check the image on the screen for subtle differences between healthy and diseased areas, decide which images to include in the report to the physician and judge whether the images are satisfactory for diagnostic purposes. They also explain the procedure to patients, record any additional medical history the patient relates, select appropriate equipment settings and change the patient's position as necessary. (See the statement on diagnostic medical sonographers elsewhere in the *Handbook* to learn more about other sonographers.)

Those who assist physicians in the diagnosis of disorders affecting the circulation are known as *vascular technologists* or *vascular sonographers*. They perform a medical history, evaluate pulses and assess blood flow in arteries and veins by listening to the vascular flow sounds for abnormalities. Then they perform a noninvasive procedure using ultrasound instrumentation to record vascular information such as vascular blood flow, blood pressure, changes in limb volume, oxygen saturation, cerebral circulation, peripheral circulation and abdominal circulation. Many of these tests are performed during or immediately after surgery.

Technologists who use ultrasound to examine the heart chambers, valves and vessels are referred to as *cardiac sonographers*, or *echocardiographers*. They use ultrasound instrumentation to create images called echocardiograms. An echocardiogram may be performed while the patient is either resting or physically active. Technologists may administer medication to physically active patients to assess their heart function. Cardiac sonographers also may assist physicians who perform transesophageal echocardiography, which involves placing a tube in the patient's esophagus to obtain ultrasound images.

Cardiovascular technicians who obtain EKGs are known as *electrocardiograph* (or *EKG*) *technicians*. To take a basic EKG, which traces electrical impulses transmitted by the heart, technicians attach electrodes to the patient's chest, arms and legs and then manipulate switches on an EKG machine to obtain a reading. An EKG is printed out for interpretation by the physician. This test is done before most kinds of surgery or as part of a routine physical examination, especially on persons who have reached middle age or who have a history of cardiovascular problems.

EKG technicians with advanced training perform Holter monitor and stress testing. For Holter monitoring, technicians place electrodes on the patient's chest and attach a portable EKG monitor to the patient's belt. Following 24 or more hours of normal activity by the patient, the technician removes a tape from the monitor and places it in a scanner.

After checking the quality of the recorded impulses on an electronic screen, the technician usually prints the information from the tape for analysis by a physician. Physicians use the output from the scanner to diagnose heart ailments, such as heart rhythm abnormalities or problems with pacemakers.

For a treadmill stress test, EKG technicians document the patient's medical history, explain the procedure, connect the patient to an EKG monitor and obtain a baseline reading and resting blood pressure. Next, they monitor the heart's performance while the patient is walking on a treadmill, gradually increasing the treadmill's speed to observe the effect of increased exertion. Like vascular technologists and cardiac sonographers, cardiographic technicians who perform EKG, Holter monitor and stress tests are known as "noninvasive" technicians.

Some cardiovascular technologists and technicians schedule appointments, type doctors' interpretations, maintain patient files and care for equipment.

Working Conditions: Technologists and technicians generally work a 5-day, 40-hour week that may include weekends. Those in catheterization laboratories tend to work longer hours and may work evenings. They also may be on call during the night and on weekends.

Cardiovascular technologists and technicians spend a lot of time walking and standing. Heavy lifting may be involved to move equipment or transfer patients. These workers wear heavy protective aprons while conducting some procedures. Those who work in catheterization laboratories may face stressful working conditions because they are in close contact with patients with serious heart ailments. For example, some patients may encounter complications that have life-or-death implications.

Training, Other Qualifications and Advancement: Although a few cardiovascular technologists, vascular technologists and cardiac sonographers are currently trained on the job, most receive training in 2- to 4-year programmes. The majority of technologists complete a 2-year junior or community college programme, but 4-year programmes are increasingly available. The first year is dedicated to core courses and is followed by a year of specialized instruction in either invasive, noninvasive cardiovascular, or noninvasive vascular technology. Those who are qualified in an allied health profession need to complete only the year of specialized instruction.

Graduates of the 33 programmes accredited by the Joint Review Committee on Education in Cardiovascular Technology are eligible to obtain professional certification in cardiac catheterization, echocardiography, vascular ultrasound and cardiographic techniques from Cardiovascular Credentialing International. Cardiac sonographers and vascular technologists also may obtain certification from the American Registry of Diagnostic Medical Sonographers.

Most EKG technicians are trained on the job by an EKG supervisor or a cardiologist. On-the-job training usually lasts about 8 to 16 weeks. Most employers prefer to train people already in the health care field—nursing aides, for example. Some EKG technicians are students enrolled in 2-year programmes to become technologists, working part time to gain experience and make contact with employers. One-year certification programmes exist for basic EKGs, Holter monitoring and stress testing. Cardiovascular technologists and technicians must be reliable, have mechanical aptitude and be able to follow detailed instructions. A pleasant, relaxed manner for putting patients at ease is an asset.

Employment: Cardiovascular technologists and technicians held about 45,000 jobs in 2004. About 3 out 4 jobs were in hospitals (private and government), primarily in cardiology departments. The remaining jobs were mostly in offices of physicians, including cardiologists or in medical and diagnostic laboratories, including diagnostic imaging centres.

Job Outlook: Employment of cardiovascular technologists and technicians is expected to grow much faster than the average for all occupations through the year 2014. Growth will occur as the population ages, because older people have a higher incidence of heart problems and use more diagnostic imaging.

Employment of vascular technologists and echocardiographers will grow as advances in vascular technology and sonography reduce the need for more costly and invasive procedures. However, fewer EKG technicians will be needed, as hospitals train nursing aides and others to perform basic EKG procedures. Individuals trained in Holter monitoring and stress testing are expected to have more favourable job prospects than are those who can perform only a basic EKG.

Some job openings for cardiovascular technologists and technicians will arise from replacement needs as individuals transfer to other jobs or leave the labour force. However, job growth and replacement needs will produce relatively few job openings because the occupation is small.

Earnings: Median annual earnings of cardiovascular technologists and technicians were $38,690 in May 2004. The middle 50 percent earned between $27,890 and $50,130. The lowest 10 percent earned less than $21,790 and the highest 10 percent earned more than $59,000. Median annual earnings of cardiovascular technologists and technicians in May 2004 were $36,890 in offices of physicians and $38,150 in general medical and surgical hospitals.

Diagnostic Medical Sonographers

Significant Points: Job opportunities should be favourable, as sonography becomes an increasingly attractive alternative to radiologic procedures.

About 6 out of 10 sonographers were employed by hospitals and most of the rest worked in offices of physicians or in medical and diagnostic laboratories, including diagnostic imaging centres.

Sonographers may train in hospitals, vocational-technical institutions, colleges and universities and the Armed Forces.

Nature of the Work: Diagnostic imaging embraces several procedures that aid in diagnosing ailments. Besides the familiar x-ray, another common diagnostic imaging method is magnetic resonance imaging, which uses giant magnets that create radio waves, rather than radiation, to form an image. Not all imaging technologies use ionizing radiation or radio waves, however. Sonography, or ultrasonography, is the use of sound waves to generate an image for the assessment and diagnosis of various medical conditions. Sonography usually is associated with obstetrics and the use of ultrasound imaging during pregnancy, but this technology has many other applications in the diagnosis and treatment of medical conditions.

Diagnostic medical sonographers, also known as *ultrasonographers*, use special equipment to direct non-ionizing, high frequency sound waves into areas of the patient's body. Sonographers operate the equipment, which collects reflected echoes and forms an image that may be videotaped, transmitted, or photographed for interpretation and diagnosis by a physician.

Sonographers begin by explaining the procedure to the patient and recording any medical history that may be relevant to the condition being viewed. They then select appropriate equipment settings and direct the patient to move into positions that will provide the best view. To perform the exam, sonographers use a transducer, which transmits sound waves in a cone—or rectangle-shaped beam. Although techniques vary with the area being examined, sonographers usually spread a special gel on the skin to aid the transmission of sound waves.

Viewing the screen during the scan, sonographers look for subtle visual cues that contrast healthy areas with unhealthy ones.

They decide whether the images are satisfactory for diagnostic purposes and select which ones to show to the physician. Sonographers take measurements, calculate values and analyze the results in preliminary reports for the physicians.

Diagnostic medical sonographers may specialize in obstetric and gynecologic sonography (the female reproductive system), abdominal sonography (the liver, kidneys, gallbladder, spleen and pancreas), neurosonography (the brain), or breast sonography. In addition, sonographers may specialize in vascular technology or echocardiography.

Obstetric and gynecologic sonographers specialize in the study of the female reproductive system. Included in the discipline is one of the more well-known uses of sonography: examining the fetus of a pregnant woman to track the baby's growth and health.

Abdominal sonographers inspect a patient's abdominal cavity to help diagnose and treat conditions primarily involving the gallbladder, bile ducts, kidneys, liver, pancreas and spleen. Abdominal sonographers also are able to scan parts of the chest, although studies of the heart using sonography usually are done by echocardiographers.

Neurosonographers focus on the nervous system, including the brain. In neonatal care, neurosonographers study and diagnose neurological and nervous system disorders in premature infants.

They also may scan blood vessels to check for abnormalities indicating a stroke in infants diagnosed with sickle-cell anemia. Like other sonographers, neurosonographers operate transducers to perform the sonogram, but use frequencies and beam shapes different from those used by obstetric and abdominal sonographers.

Breast sonographers use sonography to study the disease in breasts. Sonography aids mammography in the detection of breast cancer. Breast sonography can also track tumours, blood supply conditions and assist in the accurate biopsy of breast tissue. Breast sonographers use high-frequency transducers, made exclusively to study breast tissue.

In addition to working directly with patients, diagnostic medical sonographers keep patient records and adjust and maintain equipment. They also may prepare work schedules, evaluate equipment purchases, or manage a sonography or diagnostic imaging department.

Working Conditions: Most full-time sonographers work about 40 hours a week. Hospital-based sonographers may have evening and weekend hours and times when they are on call and must be ready to report to work on short notice.

Sonographers typically work in healthcare facilities that are clean and well lighted. Some travel to patients in large vans equipped with sophisticated diagnostic equipment. A growing number of sonographers work as contract employees and may perform tests at a number of different hospitals. Sonographers are on their feet for long periods and may have to lift or turn disabled patients. They work at diagnostic imaging machines, but also may perform some procedures at patients' bedsides.

Training, Other Qualifications and Advancement: There are several avenues for entry into the field of diagnostic medical sonography. Sonographers may train in hospitals, vocational-technical institutions, colleges and universities and the Armed Forces. Some training programmes prefer applicants with a background in science or experience in other healthcare professions, but also will consider high school graduates with courses in mathematics and science, as well as applicants with liberal arts backgrounds.

Colleges and universities offer formal training in both 2- and 4-year programmes, culminating in an associate or a bachelor's degree. Two-year programmes are most prevalent. Course work includes classes in anatomy, physiology, instrumentation, basic physics, patient care and medical ethics. The Commission on Accreditation for Allied Health Education Programmes accredits most formal training programmes—132 programmes in 2005.

Some healthcare workers, such as obstetric nurses and radiologic technologists, increase their marketability by seeking training in fields such as sonography. This usually requires completion of an additional 1-year programme that may result in a certificate. In addition, sonographers specializing in one particular discipline often seek competency in others; for example, obstetric sonographers might seek training in abdominal sonography to broaden their opportunities.

Although no State requires licensure in diagnostic medical sonography, organizations such as the American Registry for Diagnostic Medical Sonography (ARDMS) certify the competency of sonographers through registration. Because registration provides an independent, objective measure of an individual's professional standing, many employers prefer to hire registered sonographers. Registration with ARDMS requires passing a general physical principles and instrumentation examination, in addition to passing an exam in a speciality such as obstetric and gynecologic sonography, abdominal sonography, or neurosonography. To keep their registration current, sonographers must complete continuing education to stay abreast of technological advances related to the occupation.

Sonographers need good communication and interpersonal skills because they must be able to explain technical procedures and results to their patients, some of whom may be nervous about the exam or the problems it may reveal. Sonographers also should have a background in mathematics and science.

Employment: Diagnostic medical sonographers held about 42,000 jobs in 2004. About 6 out of 10 sonographer jobs were in hospitals—public and private. Most of the rest were in offices of physicians or in medical and diagnostic laboratories, including diagnostic imaging centres.

Job Outlook: Employment of diagnostic medical sonographers is expected to grow much faster than the average for all occupations through 2014 as the population grows and ages, increasing the demand for diagnostic imaging and therapeutic technology. In addition to job openings from growth, some job openings will arise from the need to replace sonographers who leave the occupation permanently.

Opportunities should be favourable because sonography is becoming an increasingly attractive alternative to radiologic procedures, as patients seek safer treatment methods. Unlike most diagnostic imaging methods, sonography does not involve radiation, so harmful side effects and complications from repeated use are rarer for both the patient and the sonographer. Sonographic technology is expected to evolve rapidly and to spawn many new sonography procedures, such as 3D- and 4D-sonography for use in obstetric and ophthalmologic diagnosis. However, high costs may limit the rate at which some promising new technologies are adopted.

Hospitals will remain the principal employer of diagnostic medical sonographers. However, employment is expected to grow more rapidly in offices of physicians and in medical and diagnostic laboratories, including diagnostic imaging centres. Healthcare facilities such as these are expected to grow very rapidly through 2014 because of the strong shift toward outpatient care, encouraged by third-party payers and made possible by technological advances that permit more procedures to be performed outside the hospital.

Earnings: Median annual earnings of diagnostic medical sonographers were $52,490 in May 2004. The middle 50 percent earned between $44,720 and $61,360 a year. The lowest 10 percent earned less than $37,800 and the highest 10 percent earned more than $72,230. Median annual earnings of diagnostic medical sonographers in May 2004 were $53,790 in offices of physicians and $51,860 in general medical and surgical hospitals.

Clinical Laboratory Technologists and Technicians

Significant Points: Faster than average employment growth is expected as the volume of laboratory tests continues to increase with both population growth and the development of new types of tests.

Clinical laboratory technologists usually have a bachelor's degree with a major in medical technology or in one of the life sciences; clinical laboratory technicians generally need either an associate degree or a certificate.

Job opportunities are expected to be excellent.

Nature of the Work: Clinical laboratory testing plays a crucial role in the detection, diagnosis and treatment of disease. Clinical laboratory technologists, also referred to as clinical laboratory scientists or medical technologists and clinical laboratory technicians, also known as medical technicians or medical laboratory technicians, perform most of these tests.

Clinical laboratory personnel examine and analyze body fluids and cells. They look for bacteria, parasites and other microorganisms; analyze the chemical content of fluids; match blood for transfusions; and test for drug levels in the blood to show how a patient is responding to treatment. Technologists also prepare specimens for examination, count cells and look for abnormal cells in blood and body fluids. They use automated equipment and computerized instruments capable of performing a number of tests simultaneously, as well as microscopes, cell counters and other sophisticated laboratory equipment. Then they analyze the results and relay them to physicians. With increasing automation and the use of computer technology, the work of technologists and technicians has become less hands-on and more analytical.

The complexity of tests performed, the level of judgment needed and the amount of responsibility workers assume depend largely on the amount of education and experience they have.

Clinical laboratory technologists perform complex chemical, biological, hematological, immunologic, microscopic and bacteriological tests. Technologists microscopically examine blood and other body fluids. They make cultures of body fluid and tissue samples, to determine the presence of bacteria, fungi, parasites, or other microorganisms. Clinical laboratory technologists analyze samples for chemical content or a chemical reaction and determine concentrations of compounds such as blood glucose and cholesterol levels. They also type and cross match blood samples for transfusions.

Clinical laboratory technologists evaluate test results, develop and modify procedures and establish and monitor programmes, to ensure the accuracy of tests. Some technologists supervise clinical laboratory technicians.

Technologists in small laboratories perform many types of tests, whereas those in large laboratories generally specialize. Technologists who prepare specimens and analyze the chemical and hormonal contents of body fluids are called clinical chemistry technologists. Those who examine and identify bacteria and other microorganisms are microbiology technologists. Blood bank technologists, or immunohematology technologists, collect, type and prepare blood and its components for transfusions. Immunology technologists examine elements of the human immune system and its response to foreign bodies. Cytotechnologists prepare slides of body cells and examine these cells microscopically for abnormalities that may signal the beginning of a cancerous growth. Molecular biology technologists perform complex protein and nucleic acid testing on cell samples.

Clinical laboratory technicians perform less complex tests and laboratory procedures than technologists perform. Technicians may prepare specimens and operate automated analyzers, for example, or they may perform manual tests in accordance with detailed instructions. Like technologists, they may work in several areas of the clinical laboratory or specialize in just one. Histotechnicians cut and stain tissue specimens for microscopic examination by pathologists and phlebotomists collect blood samples. They usually work under the supervision of medical and clinical laboratory technologists or laboratory managers.

Working Conditions: Hours and other working conditions of clinical laboratory technologists and technicians vary with the size and type of employment setting. In large hospitals or in independent laboratories that operate continuously, personnel usually work the day, evening, or night shift and may work weekends and holidays. Laboratory personnel in small facilities may work on rotating shifts, rather than on a regular shift. In some facilities, laboratory personnel are on call several nights a week or on weekends, in case of an emergency.

Clinical laboratory personnel are trained to work with infectious specimens. When proper methods of infection control and sterilization are followed, few hazards exist. Protective masks, gloves and goggles are often necessary to ensure the safety of laboratory personnel.

Laboratories usually are well lighted and clean; however, specimens, solutions and reagents used in the laboratory sometimes produce fumes. Laboratory workers may spend a great deal of time on their feet.

Training, Other Qualifications and Advancement: The usual requirement for an entry-level position as a clinical laboratory technologist is a bachelor's degree with a major in medical technology or in one of the life sciences; although it is possible to qualify through a combination of education, on-the-job and specialized training. Universities and hospitals offer medical technology programmes.

Bachelor's degree programmes in medical technology include courses in chemistry, biological sciences, microbiology, mathematics and statistics, as well as specialized courses devoted to knowledge and skills used in the clinical laboratory. Many programmes also offer or require courses in management, business and computer applications. The Clinical Laboratory Improvement Act requires technologists who perform highly complex tests to have at least an associate degree.

Medical and clinical laboratory technicians generally have either an associate degree from a community or junior college or a certificate from a hospital, a vocational or technical school, or one of the U.S. Armed Forces. A few technicians learn their skills on the job.

The National Accrediting Agency for Clinical Laboratory Sciences (NAACLS) fully accredits 469 programmes for medical and clinical laboratory technologists, medical and clinical laboratory technicians, histotechnologists and histotechnicians, cytogenetic technologists and diagnostic molecular scientists. NAACLS also approves 57 programmes in phlebotomy and clinical assisting. Other nationally recognized accrediting agencies that accredit specific areas for clinical laboratory workers include the Commission on Accreditation of Allied Health Education Programmes and the Accrediting Bureau of Health Education Schools.

Some States require laboratory personnel to be licensed or registered. Information on licensure is available from State departments of health or boards of occupational licensing. Certification is a voluntary process by which a nongovernmental organization, such as a professional society or certifying agency, grants recognition to an individual whose professional competence meets prescribed standards.

Widely accepted by employers in the health care industry, certification is a prerequisite for most jobs and often is necessary for advancement. Agencies certifying medical and clinical laboratory technologists and technicians include the Board of Registry of the American Society for Clinical Pathology, the American Medical Technologists, the National Credentialing Agency for Laboratory Personnel and the Board of Registry of the American Association of Bioanalysts. These agencies have different requirements for certification and different organizational sponsors.

Clinical laboratory personnel need good analytical judgment and the ability to work under pressure. Close attention to detail is essential, because small differences or changes in test substances or numerical readouts can be crucial for patient care. Manual dexterity and normal colour vision are highly desirable. With the widespread use of automated laboratory equipment, computer skills are important. In addition, technologists in particular are expected to be good at problem solving.

Technologists may advance to supervisory positions in laboratory work or may become chief medical or clinical laboratory technologists or laboratory managers in hospitals. Manufacturers of home diagnostic testing kits and laboratory equipment and supplies seek experienced technologists to work in product development, marketing and sales. A graduate degree in medical technology, one of the biological sciences, chemistry, management, or education usually speeds advancement. A doctorate is needed to become a laboratory director; however, Federal regulation allows directors of moderately complex laboratories to have either a master's degree or a bachelor's degree, combined with the appropriate amount of training and experience. Technicians can become technologists through additional education and experience.

Employment: Clinical laboratory technologists and technicians held about 302,000 jobs in 2004. More than half of jobs were in hospitals. Most of the remaining jobs were in offices of physicians and in medical and diagnostic laboratories. A small proportion was in educational services and in all other ambulatory health care services.

Job Outlook: Job opportunities are expected to be excellent, because the number of job openings is expected to continue to exceed the number of job seekers. Employment of clinical laboratory workers is expected to grow faster than average for all occupations through the year 2014, as the volume of laboratory tests continues to increase with both population growth and the development of new types of tests.

Technological advances will continue to have two opposing effects on employment. On the one hand, new, increasingly powerful diagnostic tests will encourage additional testing and spur employment. On the other hand, research and development efforts targeted at simplifying routine testing procedures may enhance the ability of non-laboratory personnel—physicians and patients in particular—to perform tests now conducted in laboratories. Although hospitals are expected to continue to be the major employer of clinical laboratory workers, employment is expected to grow faster in medical and diagnostic laboratories, offices of physicians and all other ambulatory health care services.

Although significant, job growth will not be the only source of opportunities. As in most occupations, many openings will result from the need to replace workers who transfer to other occupations, retire, or stop working for some other reason.

Earnings: Median annual earnings of medical and clinical laboratory technologists were $45,730 in May 2004. The middle 50 percent earned between $38,740 and $54,310. The lowest 10 percent earned less than $32,240 and the highest 10 percent earned more than $63,120. Median annual earnings in the industries employing the largest numbers of medical and clinical laboratory technologists in May 2004 were as follows:

General medical and surgical hospitals	$46,020
Medical and diagnostic laboratories	45,840
Offices of physicians	41,070

Median annual earnings of medical and clinical laboratory technicians were $30,840 in May 2004. The middle 50 percent earned between $24,890 and $37,770. The lowest 10 percent earned less than $20,410 and the highest 10 percent earned more than $45,680. Median annual earnings in the industries employing the largest numbers of medical and clinical laboratory technicians in May 2004 were as follows:

Colleges, universities and professional schools	$32,410
General medical and surgical hospitals	31,830
Offices of physicians	29,620
Medical and diagnostic laboratories	29,220
Other ambulatory health care services	28,130

According to the American Society for Clinical Pathology, median hourly wages of staff clinical laboratory technologists and technicians in 2003 varied by speciality and laboratory type as follows:

Hospital

Private Clinic	Physician office laboratory		
Cytotechnoligist	$24.70	$24.07	$25.66
Histotechnologist	19.88	19.22	20.50
Medical technologist	20.40	19.00	18.00
Histotechnician	16.97	16.13	20.00
Medical laboratory technician	16.12	15.00	14.75
Phlebotomist	11.13	10.57	10.50

Medical Scientists

Significant Points: Most medical scientists work in research and development.

Most medical scientists need a Ph.D. degree in a biological science; however, epidemiologists typically require a master's degree in public health or, in some cases, a Ph.D. or medical degree.

Despite projected rapid job growth, competition is expected for most positions.

Nature of the Work: Medical scientists research human diseases in order to improve human health. Most medical scientists conduct biomedical research and development to advance knowledge of life processes and living organisms, including viruses, bacteria and other infectious agents. Past research has resulted in advances in diagnosis, treatment and prevention of many diseases. Basic medical research continues to provide the building blocks necessary to develop solutions to human health problems, such as vaccines and medicines. Medical scientists also engage in clinical investigation, technical writing, drug application review, patent examination and related activities.

Medical scientists study biological systems to understand the causes of disease and other health problems and to develop treatments and research tools and techniques, many of which have medical applications. These scientists try to identify changes in a cell or in chromosomes that signal the development of medical problems, such as different types of cancer. For example, medical scientists involved in cancer research may formulate a combination of drugs that will lessen the effects of the disease.

Medical scientists who are also physicians can administer these drugs to patients in clinical trials, monitor their reactions and observe the results. Those who are not physicians normally collaborate with a physician who deals directly with patients. Medical scientists examine the results of clinical trials and, if necessary, adjust the dosage levels to reduce negative side effects or to try to induce even better results. In addition to developing treatments for health problems, medical scientists attempt to discover ways to prevent health problems, for example, by affirming the link between smoking and lung cancer or between alcoholism and liver disease.

Many medical scientists work independently in private industry, university, or government laboratories, often exploring new areas of research or expanding on specialized research that they began in graduate school. Medical scientists working in colleges and universities, hospitals and nonprofit medical research organizations typically submit grant proposals to obtain funding for their projects. Colleges and universities, private industry and Federal Government agencies, such as the National Institutes of Health and the National Science Foundation, contribute greatly to the support of scientists whose research proposals are determined to be financially feasible and to have the potential to advance new ideas or processes.

Medical scientists who work in applied research or product development use knowledge discovered through basic research to develop new drugs and medical treatments. They usually have less autonomy than basic medical researchers to choose the emphasis of their research, relying instead on market-driven forces arising from their firm's products and goals. Medical scientists doing applied research and product development in private industry may be required to express their research plans or results to nonscientists who are in a position to reject or approve their ideas; thus, they must understand the impact of their work on business. Scientists increasingly work as part of teams, interacting with engineers, scientists of other disciplines, business managers and technicians.

Medical scientists who conduct research usually work in laboratories and use electron microscopes, computers, thermal cyclers, or a wide variety of other equipment. Some may work directly with individual patients or larger groups as they administer drugs and monitor and observe the patients during clinical trials. Medical scientists who are also physicians may administer gene therapy to human patients, draw blood, excise tissue, or perform other invasive procedures.

Some medical scientists work in managerial, consulting, or administrative positions, usually after spending some time doing research and learning about the firm, agency, or project. In the 1980s, swift advances in basic medical knowledge related to genetics and molecules spurred growth in the field of biotechnology. Medical scientists using this technology manipulate the genetic material of animals, attempting to make organisms more productive or resistant to disease. Research using biotechnology techniques, such as recombining DNA, has led to the discovery of important drugs, including human insulin and growth hormone. Many other substances not previously available in large quantities are now produced by biotechnological means; some may one day be useful in treating diseases such as Parkinson's or Alzheimer's.

Today, many medical scientists are involved in the science of genetic engineering—isolating, identifying and sequencing human genes and then determining their function. This work continues to lead to the discovery of the genes associated with specific diseases and inherited traits, such as certain types of cancer or obesity. These advances in biotechnology have opened up research opportunities in almost all areas of medical science.

Some medical scientists specialize in epidemiology. This branch of medical science investigates and describes the determinants of disease, disability and other health outcomes and develops the means for prevention and control. Epidemiologists may study many different diseases, such as tuberculosis, influenza, or cholera, often focusing on epidemics.

Epidemiologists can be separated into two groups—research and clinical. Research epidemiologists conduct research in an effort to eradicate or control infectious diseases that affect the entire body, such as AIDS or typhus. Others may focus only on localized infections of the brain, lungs, or digestive tract, for example. Research epidemiologists work at colleges and universities, schools of public health, medical schools and research and development services firms. For example, Federal Government agencies, such as the U.S. Department of Defense, may contract with a research firm's epidemiologists to evaluate the incidence of malaria in certain parts of the world. While some perform consulting services, other research epidemiologists may work as college and university faculty.

Clinical epidemiologists work primarily in consulting roles at hospitals, informing the medical staff of infectious outbreaks and providing containment solutions. These epidemiologists sometimes are referred to as infection control professionals and some of them are also physicians. Epidemiologists who are not physicians often collaborate with physicians to find ways to contain diseases and outbreaks. In addition to traditional duties of studying and controlling diseases, clinical epidemiologists also may be required to develop standards and guidelines for the treatment and control of communicable diseases. Some clinical epidemiologists may work in outpatient settings.

Working Conditions: Medical scientists typically work regular hours in offices or laboratories and usually are not exposed to unsafe or unhealthy conditions. However, those scientists who work with dangerous organisms or toxic substances in the laboratory must follow strict safety procedures to avoid contamination. Medical scientists also spend time working in clinics and hospitals administering drugs and treatments to patients in clinical trials. On occasion, epidemiologists may be required to work evenings and weekends to attend meetings and hearings for medical investigations.

Some medical scientists depend on grant money to support their research. They may be under pressure to meet deadlines and to conform to rigid grant-writing specifications when preparing proposals to seek new or extended funding.

Training, Other Qualifications and Advancement: A Ph.D. degree in a biological science is the minimum education required for most prospective medical scientists, except epidemiologists, because the work of medical scientists is almost entirely research oriented. A Ph.D. degree qualifies one to do research on basic life processes or on particular medical problems or diseases and to analyze and interpret the results of experiments on patients. Some medical scientists obtain a medical degree instead of a Ph.D., but may not be licensed physicians because they have not taken the State licensing examination or completed a residency programme, typically because they prefer research to clinical practice.

Medical scientists who administer drug or gene therapy to human patients, or who otherwise interact medically with patients—drawing blood, excising tissue, or performing other invasive procedures—must be licensed physicians. To be licensed, physicians must graduate from an accredited medical school, pass a licensing examination and complete 1 to 7 years of graduate medical education. It is particularly helpful for medical scientists to earn both Ph.D. and medical degrees.

Students planning careers as medical scientists should have a bachelor's degree in a biological science. In addition to required courses in chemistry and biology, undergraduates should study allied disciplines, such as mathematics, engineering, physics and computer science, or courses in their field of interest. Once they have completed undergraduate studies, they can then select a speciality area for their advanced degree, such as cytology, bio-informatics, genomics, or pathology.

In addition to formal education, medical scientists usually spend several years in a postdoctoral position before they apply for permanent jobs. Postdoctoral work provides valuable laboratory experience, including experience in specific processes and techniques such as gene splicing, which is transferable to other research projects. In some institutions, the postdoctoral position can lead to a permanent job.

Medical scientists should be able to work independently or as part of a team and be able to communicate clearly and concisely, both orally and in writing. Those in private industry, especially those who aspire to consulting and administrative positions, should possess strong communication skills so that they can provide instruction and advice to physicians and other health care professionals.

The minimum educational requirement for epidemiology is a master's degree from a school of public health. Some jobs require a Ph.D. or medical degree, depending on the work performed. Epidemiologists who work in hospitals and health care centres often must have a medical degree with specific training in infectious diseases.

Currently, about 140 infectious disease training programmes exist in 42 States. Some employees in research epidemiology positions are required to be licensed physicians because they must administer drugs in clinical trials.

Epidemiologists who perform laboratory tests often require the knowledge and expertise of a licensed physician in order to administer drugs to patients in clinical trials. Epidemiologists who are not physicians frequently work closely with one.

Few students select epidemiology for undergraduate study. Undergraduates, nonetheless, should study biological sciences and should have a solid background in chemistry, mathematics and computer science. Once a student is prepared for graduate studies, he or she can choose a speciality within epidemiology. For example, those interested in studying environmental epidemiology should focus on environmental coursework, such as water pollution, air pollution, or pesticide use.

The core work of environmental studies includes toxicology and molecular biology and students may continue with advanced coursework in environmental or occupational epidemiology. Other speciality areas that students can pursue include infectious process, infection control precautions, surveillance methodology and outbreak investigation. Some epidemiologists begin their careers in other health care occupations, such as registered nurse and medical technologist..

The Association for Professionals in Infection Control and Epidemiology (APIC) offers continuing-education courses and certification programmes in infection prevention and control and applied epidemiology. To become certified as an infection control professional, applicants are required by a certified board to pass an examination for a one-time fee. Certification is recommended for those seeking advancement and for those seeking to continually upgrade their knowledge in a rapidly evolving field.

Employment: Medical scientists held about 77,000 jobs in 2004. Epidemiologists accounted for only 4,800 of that total. In addition, many medical scientists held faculty positions in colleges and universities, but they are classified as college or university faculty.

About 24 percent of medical scientists were employed in government; 24 percent were employed in scientific research and development services firms; 14 percent were employed in pharmaceutical and medicine manufacturing; 9 percent were employed in private hospitals; and most of the remainder were employed in private educational services and ambulatory health care services.

Among epidemiologists, 50 percent were employed in government; 23 percent were employed in management, scientific and technical consulting services; 12 percent were employed in scientific research and development services; and 8 percent were employed in private hospitals.

Job Outlook: Employment of medical scientists is expected to grow much faster than average for all occupations through 2014. Despite projected rapid job growth, doctoral degree holders can expect to face considerable competition for basic research positions. The Federal Government funds much basic research and development, including many areas of medical research. Recent budget increases at the National Institutes of Health have led to large increases in Federal basic research and development expenditures, with the number of grants awarded to researchers growing in number and dollar amount.

However, the increase in expenditures is expected to slow significantly over the 2004-14 projection period, resulting in a highly competitive environment for winning and renewing research grants. In addition, if the number of advanced degrees awarded continues to grow, applicants are likely to face even more competition.

Medical scientists enjoyed rapid gains in employment between the mid-1980s and mid-1990s—reflecting, in part, increased staffing requirements in new biotechnology companies. Job growth should be dampened somewhat as increases in the number of new biotechnology firms slow down and as existing firms merge or are absorbed by larger, more established biotechnology or pharmaceutical firms.

However, much of the basic medical research done in recent years has resulted in new knowledge, including the isolation and identification of new genes. Medical scientists will be needed to take this knowledge to the next stage—understanding how certain genes function within an entire organism—so that gene therapies can be developed to treat diseases. Even pharmaceutical and other firms not solely engaged in biotechnology are expected to increasingly use biotechnology techniques, thus creating employment for medical scientists.

Expected expansion in research related to health issues such as AIDS, cancer and Alzheimer's disease, along with treating growing threats such as the increase in antibiotic resistance, also should result in employment growth. Moreover, environmental conditions such as overcrowding and the increasing frequency of international travel will tend to spread existing diseases and give rise to new ones. Medical scientists will continue to be needed because they greatly contribute to the development of many treatments and medicines that improve human health.

Opportunities in epidemiology also should be highly competitive, as the number of available positions remains limited. However, an increasing focus on monitoring patients at hospitals and health care centres to ensure positive patient outcomes will contribute to job growth.

In addition, a heightened awareness of bio-terrorism and rare, but infectious diseases such as West Nile Virus or severe acute respiratory syndrome (SARS) should spur demand for these workers. As hospitals enhance their infection control programmes, many will seek to boost the quality and quantity of their staff. Besides job openings due to employment growth, additional openings will result as workers leave the labour force or transfer to other occupations.

Medical scientists and some epidemiologists are less likely to lose their jobs during recessions than are those in many other occupations because they are employed on long-term research projects. However, a recession could influence the amount of money allocated to new research and development, particularly in areas of risky or innovative medical research. A recession also could limit extensions or renewals of existing projects.

Earnings: Median annual earnings of medical scientists, except epidemiologists, were $61,320 in May 2004. The middle 50 percent of these workers earned between $44,120 and $86,830. The lowest 10 percent earned less than $33,030 and the highest 10 percent earned more than $114,360. Median annual earnings in the industries employing the largest numbers of medical scientists in May 2004 were:

Pharmaceutical and medicine manufacturing	$76,800
Scientific research and development services	65,110
General medical and surgical hospitals	55,410
Colleges, universities and professional schools	45,600

Median annual earnings of epidemiologists were $54,800 in May 2004. The middle 50 percent earned between $45,320 and $67,160. The lowest 10 percent earned less than $36,130 and the highest 10 percent earned more than $82,310.

Dentists

Significant Points: Most dentists are solo practitioners.

Dentists usually complete at least 8 years of education beyond high school.

Employment is projected to grow about as fast as average and most job openings will result from the need to replace the large number of dentists expected to retire.

Job prospects should be good.

Nature of the Work: Dentists diagnose, prevent and treat problems with teeth or mouth tissue. They remove decay, fill cavities, examine x rays, place protective plastic sealants on children's teeth, straighten teeth and repair fractured teeth. They also perform corrective surgery on gums and supporting bones to treat gum diseases. Dentists extract teeth and make models and measurements for dentures to replace missing teeth. They provide instruction on diet, brushing, flossing, the use of fluorides and other aspects of dental care. They also administer anesthetics and write prescriptions for antibiotics and other medications.

Dentists use a variety of equipment, including x-ray machines; drills; and instruments such as mouth mirrors, probes, forceps, brushes and scalpels. They wear masks, gloves and safety glasses to protect themselves and their patients from infectious diseases.

Dentists in private practice oversee a variety of administrative tasks, including bookkeeping and buying equipment and supplies. They may employ and supervise dental hygienists, dental assistants, dental laboratory technicians and receptionists.

Most dentists are general practitioners, handling a variety of dental needs. Other dentists practice in any of nine speciality areas. *Orthodontists*, the largest group of specialists, straighten teeth by applying pressure to the teeth with braces or retainers. The next largest group, *oral and maxillofacial surgeons*, operates on the mouth and jaws.

The remainder may specialize as *pediatric dentists* (focusing on dentistry for children); *periodontists* (treating gums and bone supporting the teeth); *prosthodontists* (replacing missing teeth with permanent fixtures, such as crowns and bridges, or with removable fixtures such as dentures); *endodontists* (performing root canal therapy); *public health dentists* (promoting good dental health and preventing dental diseases within the community); *oral pathologists* (studying oral diseases); or *oral and maxillofacial radiologists* (diagnosing diseases in the head and neck through the use of imaging technologies).

Working Conditions: Most dentists work 4 or 5 days a week. Some work evenings and weekends to meet their patients' needs. Most full-time dentists work between 35 and 40 hours a week, but others work more.

Initially, dentists may work more hours as they establish their practice. Experienced dentists often work fewer hours. Many continue in part-time practice well beyond the usual retirement age.

Most dentists are solo practitioners, meaning that they own their own businesses and work alone or with a small staff. Some dentists have partners and a few work for other dentists as associate dentists.

Training, Other Qualifications and Advancement: All 50 States and the District of Columbia require dentists to be licensed. To qualify for a license in most States, candidates must graduate from 1 of the 56 dental schools accredited by the American Dental Association's (ADA's) Commission on Dental Accreditation in 2004 and then must pass written and practical examinations. Candidates may fulfil the written part of the State licensing requirements by passing the National Board Dental Examinations. Individual States or regional testing agencies administer the written or practical examinations.

Dental schools require a minimum of 2 years of college-level predental education, regardless of the major chosen. However, most dental students have at least a bachelor's degree. Predental education emphasizes coursework in science and many applicants to dental school major in a science such as biology or chemistry, while other applicants major in another subject and take many science courses as well. A few applicants are accepted to dental school after 2 or 3 years of college and complete their bachelor's degree while attending dental school.

All dental schools require applicants to take the Dental Admissions Test (DAT). When selecting students, schools consider scores earned on the DAT, applicants' grade point averages and information gathered through recommendations and interviews. Competition for admission to dental school is keen.

Dental school usually lasts 4 academic years. Studies begin with classroom instruction and laboratory work in basic sciences, including anatomy, microbiology, biochemistry and physiology. Beginning courses in clinical sciences, including laboratory techniques, also are provided at this time. During the last 2 years, students treat patients, usually in dental clinics, under the supervision of licensed dentists. Most dental schools award the degree of Doctor of Dental Surgery (DDS). The rest award an equivalent degree, Doctor of Dental Medicine (DMD).

Some dental school graduates work for established dentists as associates for 1 to 2 years to gain experience and save money to equip an office of their own. Most dental school graduates, however, purchase an established practice or open a new one immediately after graduation.

In 2004, 17 States licensed or certified dentists who intended to practice in a speciality area. Requirements include 2 to 4 years of postgraduate education and, in some cases, the completion of a special State examination. Most State licenses permit dentists to engage in both general and specialized practice.

Dentists who want to teach or conduct research usually spend an additional 2 to 5 years in advanced dental training, in programmes operated by dental schools or hospitals. According to the ADA, each year about 12 percent of new graduates enrol in postgraduate training programmes to prepare for a dental speciality.

Dentistry requires diagnostic ability and manual skills. Dentists should have good visual memory, excellent judgment regarding space and shape, a high degree of manual dexterity and scientific ability. Good business sense, self-discipline and good communication skills are helpful for success in private practice. High school and college students who want to become dentists should take courses in biology, chemistry, physics, health and mathematics.

Employment: Dentists held about 150,000 jobs in 2004. Employment was distributed among general practitioners and specialists as follows:

Dentists, general	128,000
Orthodontists	10,000
Oral and maxillofacial surgeons	6,000
Prosthodontists	1,000
Dentists, all other specialists	5,000

About one third of dentists were self-employed and not incorporated. Almost all dentists work in private practice. According to ADA, 78 percent of dentists in private practice are sole proprietors and 14 percent belong to a partnership. A few salaried dentists work in hospitals and offices of physicians.

Job Outlook: Employment of dentists is projected to grow about as fast as average for all occupations through 2014. Although employment growth will provide some job opportunities, most jobs will result from the need to replace the large number of dentists expected to retire. Job prospects should be good as new dentists take over established practices or start their own.

Demand for dental care should grow substantially through 2014. As members of the baby-boom generation advance into middle age, a large number will need complicated dental work, such as bridges. In addition, elderly people are more likely to retain their teeth than were their predecessors, so they will require much more care than in the past. The younger generation will continue to need preventive checkups despite treatments such as fluoridation of the water supply, which decreases the incidence of tooth decay. However, employment of dentists is not expected to grow as rapidly as the demand for dental services. As their practices expand, dentists are likely to hire more dental hygienists and dental assistants to handle routine services.

Dentists will increasingly provide care and instruction aimed at preventing the loss of teeth, rather than simply providing treatments such as fillings. Improvements in dental technology also will allow dentists to offer more effective and less painful treatment to their patients.

Earnings: Median annual earnings of salaried dentists were $129,920 in May 2004. Earnings vary according to number of years in practice, location, hours worked and speciality.

Self-employed dentists in private practice tend to earn more than do salaried dentists and a relatively large proportion of dentists is self-employed. Like other business owners, these dentists must provide their own health insurance, life insurance and retirement benefits.

Dental Assistants

Significant Points: Job prospects should be excellent.

Dentists are expected to hire more assistants to perform routine tasks so that they may devote their own time to more complex procedures.

Most assistants learn their skills on the job, although an increasing number are trained in dental-assisting programmes; most programmes take 1 year or less to complete.

Nature of the Work: Dental assistants perform a variety of patient care, office and laboratory duties. They work chairside as dentists examine and treat patients. They make patients as comfortable as possible in the dental chair, prepare them for treatment and obtain their dental records.

Assistants hand instruments and materials to dentists and keep patients' mouths dry and clear by using suction or other devices. Assistants also sterilize and disinfect instruments and equipment, prepare trays of instruments for dental procedures and instruct patients on postoperative and general oral health care.

Some dental assistants prepare materials for impressions and restorations, take dental x rays and process x-ray film as directed by a dentist. They also may remove sutures, apply topical anesthetics to gums or cavity-preventive agents to teeth, remove excess cement used in the filling process and place rubber dams on the teeth to isolate them for individual treatment.

Those with laboratory duties make casts of the teeth and mouth from impressions, clean and polish removable appliances and make temporary crowns. Dental assistants with office duties schedule and confirm appointments, receive patients, keep treatment records, send bills, receive payments and order dental supplies and materials.

Dental assistants should not be confused with dental hygienists, who are licensed to perform different clinical tasks.

Working Conditions: Dental assistants work in a well-lighted, clean environment. Their work area usually is near the dental chair so that they can arrange instruments, materials and medication and hand them to the dentist when needed. Dental assistants must wear gloves, masks, eyewear and protective clothing to protect themselves and their patients from infectious diseases.

Assistants also follow safety procedures to minimize the risks associated with the use of x-ray machines.

About half of dental assistants have a 35- to 40-hour workweek, which may include work on Saturdays or evenings.

Training, Other Qualifications and Advancement: Most assistants learn their skills on the job, although an increasing number are trained in dental-assisting programmes offered by community and junior colleges, trade schools, technical institutes, or the Armed Forces. Assistants must be a second pair of hands for a dentist; therefore, dentists look for people who are reliable, work well with others and have good manual dexterity. High school students interested in a career as a dental assistant should take courses in biology, chemistry, health and office practices.

The Commission on Dental Accreditation within the American Dental Association (ADA) approved 265 dental-assisting training programmes in 2005. Programmes include classroom, laboratory and preclinical instruction in dental-assisting skills and related theory. In addition, students gain practical experience in dental schools, clinics, or dental offices. Most programmes take 1 year or less to complete and lead to a certificate or diploma. Two-year programmes offered in community and junior colleges lead to an associate degree. All programmes require a high school diploma or its equivalent and some require science or computer-related courses for admission. A number of private vocational schools offer 4-month to 6-month courses in dental assisting, but the Commission on Dental Accreditation does not accredit these programmes.

Most States regulate the duties that dental assistants are allowed to perform through licensure or registration. Licensure or registration may require passing a written or practical examination. States offering licensure or registration have a variety of schools offering courses—approximately 10 to 12 months in length—that meet their State's requirements. Other States require dental assistants to complete State-approved education courses of 4 to 12 hours in length. Some States offer registration of other dental assisting credentials with little or no education required. Some States require continuing education to maintain licensure or registration. A few States allow dental assistants to perform any function delegated to them by the dentist.

Individual States have adopted different standards for dental assistants who perform certain advanced duties, such as radiological procedures. Completion of the Radiation Health and Safety examination offered by the Dental Assisting National Board (DANB) meets those standards in more than 30 States. Some States require completion of a State-approved course in radiology as well.

Certification is available through DANB and is recognized or required in more than 30 States. Other organizations offer registration, most often at the State level. Certification is an acknowledgment of an assistant's qualifications and professional competence and may be an asset when one is seeking employment. Candidates may qualify to take the DANB certification examination by graduating from an ADA-accredited dental assisting education programme or by having 2 years of full-time, or 4 years of part-time, experience as a dental assistant. In addition, applicants must have current certification in cardiopulmonary resuscitation. For annual recertification, individuals must earn continuing education credits.

Without further education, advancement opportunities are limited. Some dental assistants become office managers, dental-assisting instructors, or dental product sales representatives. Others go back to school to become dental hygienists. For many, this entry-level occupation provides basic training and experience and serves as a stepping-stone to more highly skilled and higher paying jobs.

Employment: Dental assistants held about 267,000 jobs in 2004. Almost all jobs for dental assistants were in offices of dentists. A small number of jobs were in the Federal, State and local governments or in offices of physicians. About 2 out of 5 dental assistants worked part time, sometimes in more than one dental office.

Job Outlook: Job prospects for dental assistants should be excellent. Employment is expected to grow much faster than average for all occupations through the year 2014. In fact, dental assistants is expected to be one of the fastest growing occupations over the 2004-14 projection period.

In addition to job openings due to employment growth, numerous job openings will arise out of the need to replace assistants who transfer to other occupations, retire, or leave for other reasons. Many opportunities are for entry-level positions offering on-the-job training.

Population growth and greater retention of natural teeth by middle-aged and older people will fuel demand for dental services. Older dentists, who have been less likely to employ assistants, are leaving the occupation and will be replaced by recent graduates, who are more likely to use one or even two assistants. In addition, as dentists' workloads increase, they are expected to hire more assistants to perform routine tasks, so that they may devote their own time to more complex procedures.

Earnings: Median hourly earnings of dental assistants were $13.62 in May 2004. The middle 50 percent earned between $11.06 and $16.65 an hour. The lowest 10 percent earned less than $9.11 and the highest 10 percent earned more than $19.97 an hour.

Benefits vary substantially by practice setting and may be contingent upon full-time employment. According to the American Dental Association (ADA), almost all full-time dental assistants employed by private practitioners received paid vacation time. The ADA also found that 9 out of 10 full-time and part-time dental assistants received dental coverage.

Podiatrists

Significant Points: Despite increasing demand for podiatric care, job openings for podiatrists are expected to be limited because the occupation is small and most podiatrists remain in it until they retire.

Opportunities for newly trained podiatrists will be better in group medical practices, clinics and health networks than in traditional, solo practices.

Podiatrists need a State license that requires the completion of at least 90 hours of undergraduate study; a 4-year postgraduate programme at a college of podiatric medicine; and, in most States, a postdoctoral residency programme lasting at least 2 years.

Podiatrists enjoy very high earnings.

Nature of the Work: Americans spend a great deal of time on their feet. As the Nation becomes more active across all age groups, the need for foot care will become increasingly important to maintaining a healthy lifestyle.

The human foot is a complex structure. It contains 26 bones—plus muscles, nerves, ligaments and blood vessels—and is designed for balance and mobility. The 52 bones in the feet make up about one-fourth of all the bones in the human body. Podiatrists, also known as *doctors of podiatric medicine* (DPMs), diagnose and treat disorders, diseases and injuries of the foot and lower leg.

Podiatrists treat corns, calluses, ingrown toenails, bunions, heel spurs and arch problems; ankle and foot injuries, deformities and infections; and foot complaints associated with diseases such as diabetes. To treat these problems, podiatrists prescribe drugs, order physical therapy, set fractures and perform surgery. They also fit corrective inserts called orthotics, design plaster casts and strappings to correct deformities and design custom-made shoes. Podiatrists may use a force plate or scanner to help design the orthotics: patients walk across a plate connected to a computer that "reads" their feet, picking up pressure points and weight distribution. From the computer readout, podiatrists order the correct design or recommend another kind of treatment.

To diagnose a foot problem, podiatrists also order x rays and laboratory tests. The foot may be the first area to show signs of serious conditions such as arthritis, diabetes and heart disease. For example, patients with diabetes are prone to foot ulcers and infections due to poor circulation. Podiatrists consult with and refer patients to other health practitioners when they detect symptoms of these disorders.

Most podiatrists have a solo practice, although more are forming group practices with other podiatrists or health practitioners. Some specialize in surgery, orthopedics, primary care, or public health. Besides these board-certified specialities, podiatrists may practice other specialities, such as sports medicine, pediatrics, dermatology, radiology, geriatrics, or diabetic foot care.

Podiatrists who are in private practice are responsible for running a small business. They may hire employees, order supplies and keep records, among other tasks. In addition, some educate the community on the benefits of foot care through speaking engagements and advertising.

Working Conditions: Podiatrists usually work in their own offices. They also may spend time visiting patients in nursing homes or performing surgery at hospitals or ambulatory surgical centres, but usually have fewer afterhours emergencies than other doctors have. Those with private practices set their own hours, but may work evenings and weekends to accommodate their patients.

Training, Other Qualifications and Advancement: All States and the District of Columbia require a license for the practice of podiatric medicine. Each State defines its own licensing requirements, although many States grant reciprocity to podiatrists who are licensed in another State. Applicants for licensure must be graduates of an accredited college of podiatric medicine and must pass written and oral examinations. Some States permit applicants to substitute the examination of the National Board of Podiatric Medical Examiners, given in the second and fourth years of podiatric medical college, for part or all of the written State examination. Most States also require the completion of a postdoctoral residency programme of at least 2 years and continuing education for license renewal.

Prerequisites for admission to a college of podiatric medicine include the completion of at least 90 semester hours of undergraduate study, an acceptable grade point average and suitable scores on the Medical College Admission Test (some colleges also may accept the Dental Admission Test or the Graduate Record Exam). All of the colleges require 8 semester hours each of biology, inorganic chemistry, organic chemistry and physics, as well as 6 hours of English. The science courses should be those designed for premedical students. Potential podiatric medical students also are evaluated on the basis of extracurricular and community activities, personal interviews and letters of recommendation. About 95 percent of podiatric students have at least a bachelor's degree.

In 2005, there were seven colleges of podiatric medicine accredited by the Council on Podiatric Medical Education. Colleges of podiatric medicine offer a 4-year programme whose core curriculum is similar to that in other schools of medicine. During the first 2 years, students receive classroom instruction in basic sciences, including anatomy, chemistry, pathology and pharmacology. Third- and fourth-year students have clinical rotations in private practices, hospitals and clinics. During these rotations, they learn how to take general and podiatric histories, perform routine physical examinations, interpret tests and findings, make diagnoses and perform therapeutic procedures. Graduates receive the degree of Doctor of Podiatric Medicine (DPM).

Most graduates complete a hospital-based residency programme after receiving a DPM. Residency programmes last from 2 to 4 years. Residents receive advanced training in podiatric medicine and surgery and serve clinical rotations in anesthesiology, internal medicine, pathology, radiology, emergency medicine and orthopedic and general surgery. Residencies lasting more than 1 year provide more extensive training in speciality areas.

There are a number of certifying boards for the podiatric specialities of orthopedics, primary medicine and surgery. Certification means that the DPM meets higher standards than those required for licensure. Each board requires advanced training, the completion of written and oral examinations and experience as a practicing podiatrist. Most managed-care organizations prefer board-certified podiatrists.

People planning a career in podiatry should have scientific aptitude, manual dexterity, interpersonal skills and good business sense. Podiatrists may advance to become professors at colleges of podiatric medicine, department chiefs in hospitals, or general health administrators.

Employment: Podiatrists held about 10,000 jobs in 2004. About 23 percent of podiatrists are self-employed. Most podiatrists were solo practitioners, although more are entering group practices with other podiatrists or other health practitioners. Solo practitioners primarily were unincorporated self-employed workers, although some also were incorporated wage and salary workers in offices of other health practitioners. Other podiatrists are employed in hospitals and by the Federal Government.

Job Outlook: Employment of podiatrists is expected to grow about as fast as average for all occupations through 2014. More people will turn to podiatrists for foot care because of the rising number of injuries sustained by a more active and increasingly older population. Additional job openings will result from podiatrists who retire from the occupation, particularly members of the baby-boom generation. However, relatively few job openings from this source are expected because the occupation is small and most podiatrists remain in it until they retire.

Medicare and most private health insurance programmes cover acute medical and surgical foot services, as well as diagnostic x rays and leg braces. Details of such coverage vary among plans. However, routine foot care, including the removal of corns and calluses, ordinarily is not covered unless the patient has a systemic condition that has resulted in severe circulatory problems or areas of desensitization in the legs or feet. Like dental services, podiatric care is often discretionary and, therefore, more dependent on disposable income than some other medical services.

Employment of podiatrists would grow even faster were it not for continued emphasis on controlling the costs of speciality health care. Insurers will balance the cost of sending patients to podiatrists against the cost and availability of substitute practitioners, such as physicians and physical therapists. Opportunities will be better for board-certified podiatrists, because many managed-care organizations require board certification. Opportunities for newly trained podiatrists will be better in group medical practices, clinics and health networks than in traditional solo practices. Establishing a practice will be most difficult in the areas surrounding colleges of podiatric medicine, where podiatrists are concentrated.

Earnings: Podiatrists enjoy very high earnings. Median annual earnings of salaried podiatrists were $94,400 in 2004.

Additionally, a survey by *Podiatry Management Magazine* reported median net income of $113,000 in 2004. Podiatrists in partnerships tended to earn higher net incomes than those in solo practice. Self-employed podiatrists must provide for their own health insurance and retirement.

Massage Therapists

Significant Points: Employment is expected to grow faster than average over the 2004-2014 period as more people learn about the benefits of massage therapy.

Many States require formal training and a national certification in order to practice massage therapy.

This occupation contains a large number of part-time and self-employed workers.

Nature of the Work: Many physicians have been recommending massage therapy for years. Nearly 2,400 years. The medical benefits of "friction" were first documented in Western culture by the Greek physician Hippocrates around 400 BC. Today, massage therapy is being used as a means of treating painful ailments, decompressing tired and overworked muscles, reducing stress, rehabilitating sports injuries and promoting general health. This is accomplished by manipulating a client's soft tissues in order to improve the body's circulation and remove waste products from the muscles.

While massage therapy is done for medical benefit, a massage can be given to simply relax or rejuvenate the person being massaged. It is important to note that this type of massage is not intended for a medical purpose and provides medical value only through general stress reduction and increased energy levels. Massage therapy, on the other hand, is practiced by thoroughly trained individuals who provide specialized care with their client's medical health in mind.

Massage therapists can specialize in over 80 different types of massage, called modalities. Swedish massage, deep tissue massage, reflexology, acupressure, sports massage and neuromuscular massage are just a few of the many approaches to massage therapy. Most massage therapists specialize in several modalities, which require different techniques. Some use exaggerated strokes ranging the length of a body part, while others use quick, percussion-like strokes with a cupped or closed hand. A massage can be as long as two hours or as short as five or ten minutes.

Usually, the type of massage therapists give depends on the client's needs and the client's physical condition. For example, they use special techniques for elderly clients that they would not use for athletes and they would use approaches for clients with injuries that would not be appropriate for clients seeking relaxation. There are also some forms of massage that are given solely to one type of client, for example prenatal massage and infant massage.

Massage therapists work by appointment. Before beginning a massage therapy session, therapists conduct an informal interview with the client to find out about the person's medical history and desired results from the massage. This gives therapists a chance to discuss which techniques could be beneficial to the client and which could be harmful. Because massage therapists tend to specialize in only a few areas of massage, customers will often be referred or seek a therapist with a certain type of massage in mind.

Based on the person's goals, ailments, medical history and stress—or pain-related problem areas, a massage therapist will conclude whether a massage would be harmful and if not, move forward with the session while concentrating on any areas of particular discomfort to the client. While giving the massage, therapists alter their approach or concentrate on a particular area as necessary.

Many modalities of massage therapy use massage oils, lotions, or creams to massage and rub the client's muscles. Most massage therapists, particularly those who are self-employed, supply their own table or chair, sheets, pillows and body lotions or oils. Most modalities of massage require clients to be covered in a sheet or blanket and require clients to be undressed or to wear loose-fitting clothing. The therapist only exposes the body part on which he or she is currently massaging. Some types of massage are done without oils or lotions and are performed with the client fully-clothed.

Massage can be a delicate issue for some clients and those clients may indicate that they are comfortable with contact only in specified areas. For this reason—and also for general purpose business risks—about half of all massage therapists have liability insurance, either through a professional association membership or through other insurance carriers.

Massage therapists must develop a rapport with their clients if repeat customers are to be secured. Because those who seek a therapist tend to make regular visits, developing a loyal clientele is an important part of becoming successful.

Working Conditions: Massage therapists work in an array of settings both private and public: private offices, studios, hospitals, nursing homes, fitness centres, sports medicine facilities, airports and shopping malls, for example. Some massage therapists also travel to clients' homes or offices to provide a massage. It is not uncommon for full-time massage therapists to divide their time among several different settings, depending on the clients and locations scheduled.

Most massage therapists give massages in dimly lit settings. Using candles and/or incense is not uncommon. Ambient or other calm, soothing music is often played. The dim lighting, smells and background noise are meant to put clients at ease. On the other hand, when visiting a client's office, a massage therapist may not have those amenities. The working conditions depend heavily on a therapist's location and what the client wants.

Because massage is physically demanding, massage therapists can succumb to injury if the proper technique is not used. Repetitive motion problems and fatigue from standing for extended periods of time are most common. This risk can be limited by use of good technique, proper spacing between sessions, exercise and in many cases by the therapists themselves receiving a massage on a regular basis.

Because of the physical nature of the work and time needed in between sessions, massage therapists typically give massages less than 40 hours per week. Therapists who give massages anywhere from 15 to 30 hours per week usually consider themselves to be full-time workers.

Training, Other Qualifications and Advancement: Training standards and requirements for massage therapists vary greatly by State and locality. In 2004, 33 States and the District of Columbia had passed laws regulating massage therapy in some way.

Most of the boards governing massage therapy in these States require practicing massage therapists to complete a formal education programme and pass the national certification examination or a State exam. Some State regulations require that therapists keep up on their knowledge and technique through continuing education. It is best to check information on licensing, certification and accreditation on a State-by-State basis.

There are roughly 1,300 massage therapy post-secondary schools, college programmes and training programmes throughout the country. Massage therapy programmes generally cover subjects such as anatomy; physiology, the study of organs and tissues; kinesiology, the study of motion and body mechanics; business; ethics; as well as hands-on practice of massage techniques. Most formal training programmes require an application and some require an in-person interview. Training programmes may concentrate on certain modalities of massage. Several programmes also provide alumni services such as postgraduate job placement and continuing educational services. Both full—and part-time programmes are available.

These programmes vary in accreditation. Massage therapy training programmes are generally accredited by a State board or other accrediting agency. Of the many massage therapy programmes in the country, about 300 are accredited by a State board or department of education-certified accrediting agency. In States that regulate massage therapy, graduation from an approved school or training programme is usually required in order to practice massage therapy.

After completion of a training programme, many massage therapists opt to take the national certification examination for therapeutic massage and bodywork. This exam is administered by the National Certification Board for Therapeutic Massage and Bodywork (NCBTMB), which has eligibility requirements of its own. Several States require that a massage therapist pass this test in order to practice massage therapy. In States that require massage therapy programme accreditation, an exam candidate must graduate from a State-licensed training institute with at least 500 hours of training or submit a portfolio of training experience for NCBTMB review; in locations that do not require accredited training programmes, this is unnecessary.

After the applicant is approved for testing, the applicant may schedule a test time at a local testing centre. Tests are available six or seven days a week, depending on the test site and are entirely computer based with multiple choice questions. The exam covers six areas of content: general knowledge of the body systems; detailed knowledge of anatomy, physiology and kinesiology; pathology; therapeutic massage assessment; therapeutic massage application; and professional standards, ethics, business and legal practices.

When a therapist passes the national certification exam for therapeutic massage and bodywork, he or she can use the recognized national credential: Nationally Certified in Therapeutic Massage and Bodywork (NCTMB). The credential must be renewed every four years.

In order to remain certified, a therapist must perform at least 200 hours of therapeutic massage during the four year period and complete a minimum of 48 credit hours of continuing education. In 2005, the NCBTMB introduced a new national certification test and corresponding professional credential. These are the national certification exam for therapeutic massage and the Nationally Certified in Therapeutic Massage (NCTM) credential. The new test covers the same topics as the traditional national certification exam, but covers fewer modalities of massage therapy. Recognition of this new national certification varies by State.

Many of the national, State and local requirements coincide. States that require the national credential also require accredited training programmes to comply with NCBTMB standards of training. Professional associations require that a professional member graduate from a training programme that meets NCBTMB standards, have a State license and/or have a national certification from the NCBTMB. Actual requirements differ on a State-by-State basis.

Because of the nature of massage therapy, opportunities for advancement are limited. However, with increased experience and an expanding client base, there are opportunities for therapists to increase client fees and therefore income.

Both strong communication skills and a friendly, empathetic personality are extremely helpful qualities for fostering a trusting relationship with clients and in turn, expanding one's client base. In addition, those who are well organized and have an entrepreneurial spirit may even go into business for themselves. Self-employed massage therapists with a large client base have the highest earnings.

Employment: Massage therapists held about 97,000 jobs in 2004. About two-thirds were self-employed. Of those self-employed, most owned their own business and the rest worked as independent contractors. Others found employment in salons and spas; the offices of physicians and chiropractors; fitness and recreational sports centres; and hotels. About three-quarters of all massage therapists worked part-time or had variable schedules, although as mentioned earlier many massage therapists who work 15 to 30 hours per week consider themselves to be full-time workers.

Job Outlook: Employment for massage therapists is expected to increase faster than average over the period from 2004 to 2014 as more people learn about the benefits of massage therapy. In States that regulate massage therapy, therapists who complete formal training programmes and pass the national certification exam are likely to have very good job opportunities. Because referrals are a very important source of work for massage therapists, networking will increase the number of job opportunities. Joining a State or local chapter of a professional association can also help build strong contacts and further increase the likelihood of steady work.

Massage is an increasingly popular technique for relaxation and reduction of stress. As workplaces try to distinguish themselves as employee-friendly, providing professional in-office, seated massages for employees is becoming a popular on-the-job benefit.

Increased interest in alternative medicine and holistic healing will mean increased opportunities for those skilled in massage therapy. Healthcare providers and medical insurance companies are beginning to recognize massage therapy as a legitimate treatment and preventative measure for several types of injuries and illnesses. The health care industry is using massage therapy more often as a supplement to conventional medical techniques for ailments such as muscle problems, some sicknesses and diseases and stress-related health problems. Massage therapy's growing acceptance as a medical tool, particularly by the medical provider and insurance industries, will greatly increase employment opportunities.

Older citizens who are in nursing homes or assisted living homes are also finding benefits from massage, such as increased energy levels and reduced health problems. Demand for massage therapy should grow among older age groups because they increasingly enjoy longer, more active lives and persons age 55 and older are projected to be the most rapidly growing segment of the U.S. population over the next decade. However, demand for massage therapy is presently greatest among young adults and they are likely to continue to enjoy the benefits of massage therapy as they age.

Earnings: Median hourly earnings of massage therapists, including gratuities earned, were $15.36 in May 2004. The middle 50 percent earned between $9.78 and $23.82. The lowest 10 percent earned less than $7.16 and the highest 10 percent earned more than $32.21. Generally, massage therapists earn 15 to 20 percent of their income as gratuities. For those who work in a hospital or other clinical setting, however, tipping is not common.

Medical Assistants

Significant Points: About 6 out of 10 medical assistants work in offices of physicians.

Some medical assistants are trained on the job, but many complete 1- or 2-year programmes in vocational-technical high schools, post-secondary vocational schools and community and junior colleges.

Medical assistants is projected to be one of the fastest growing occupations over the 2004-14 period.

Job prospects should be best for medical assistants with formal training or experience, particularly those with certification.

Nature of the Work: Medical assistants perform administrative and clinical tasks to keep the offices of physicians, podiatrists, chiropractors and other health practitioners running smoothly. They should not be confused with physician assistants, who examine, diagnose and treat patients under the direct supervision of a physician.

The duties of medical assistants vary from office to office, depending on the location and size of the practice and the practitioner's speciality. In small practices, medical assistants usually are generalists, handling both administrative and clinical duties and reporting directly to an office manager, physician, or other health practitioner.

Those in large practices tend to specialize in a particular area, under the supervision of department administrators.

Medical assistants perform many administrative duties, including answering telephones, greeting patients, updating and filing patients' medical records, filling out insurance forms, handling correspondence, scheduling appointments, arranging for hospital admission and laboratory services and handling billing and bookkeeping.

Clinical duties vary according to State law and include taking medical histories and recording vital signs, explaining treatment procedures to patients, preparing patients for examination and assisting the physician during the examination. Medical assistants collect and prepare laboratory specimens or perform basic laboratory tests on the premises, dispose of contaminated supplies and sterilize medical instruments. They instruct patients about medications and special diets, prepare and administer medications as directed by a physician, authorize drug refills as directed, telephone prescriptions to a pharmacy, draw blood, prepare patients for x rays, take electrocardiograms, remove sutures and change dressings.

Medical assistants also may arrange examining room instruments and equipment, purchase and maintain supplies and equipment and keep waiting and examining rooms neat and clean.

Ophthalmic medical assistants and *podiatric medical assistants* are examples of specialized assistants who have additional duties. Ophthalmic medical assistants help ophthalmologists provide eye care. They conduct diagnostic tests, measure and record vision and test eye muscle function. They also show patients how to insert, remove and care for contact lenses and they apply eye dressings. Under the direction of the physician, ophthalmic medical assistants may administer eye medications. They also maintain optical and surgical instruments and may assist the ophthalmologist in surgery. Podiatric medical assistants make castings of feet, expose and develop x rays and assist podiatrists in surgery.

Working Conditions: Medical assistants work in well-lighted, clean environments. They constantly interact with other people and may have to handle several responsibilities at once.

Most full-time medical assistants work a regular 40-hour week. Many work part time, evenings, or weekends.

Training, Other Qualifications and Advancement: Most employers prefer graduates of formal programmes in medical assisting. Such programmes are offered in vocational-technical high schools, post-secondary vocational schools and community and junior colleges.

Post-secondary programmes usually last either 1 year, resulting in a certificate or diploma, or 2 years, resulting in an associate degree. Courses cover anatomy, physiology and medical terminology, as well as typing, transcription, record-keeping, accounting and insurance processing. Students learn laboratory techniques, clinical and diagnostic procedures, pharmaceutical principles, the administration of medications and first aid. They study office practices, patient relations, medical law and ethics. Accredited programmes include an internship that provides practical experience in physicians' offices, hospitals, or other health care facilities.

Both the Commission on Accreditation of Allied Health Education Programmes (CAAHEP) and the Accrediting Bureau of Health Education Schools (ABHES) accredit programmes in medical assisting. In 2005, there were over 500 medical assisting programmes accredited by CAAHEP and about 170 accredited by ABHES. The Committee on Accreditation for Ophthalmic Medical Personnel approved 17 programmes in ophthalmic medical assisting and 2 programmes in ophthalmic clinical assisting.

Formal training in medical assisting, while generally preferred, is not always required. Some medical assistants are trained on the job, although this practice is less common than in the past. Applicants usually need a high school diploma or the equivalent. Recommended high school courses include mathematics, health, biology, typing, bookkeeping, computers and office skills. Volunteer experience in the health care field also is helpful.

Although medical assistants are not licensed, some States require them to take a test or a course before they can perform certain tasks, such as taking x rays or giving injections.

Employers prefer to hire experienced workers or certified applicants who have passed a national examination, indicating that the medical assistant meets certain standards of competence. The American Association of Medical Assistants awards the Certified Medical Assistant credential; American Medical Technologists awards the Registered Medical Assistant credential; the American Society of Podiatric Medical Assistants awards the Podiatric Medical Assistant, Certified credential; and the Joint Commission on Allied Health Personnel in Ophthalmology awards credentials at three levels: Certified Ophthalmic Assistant; Certified Ophthalmic Technician; and Certified Ophthalmic Medical Technologist.

Medical assistants deal with the public; therefore, they must be neat and well groomed and have a courteous, pleasant manner. Medical assistants must be able to put patients at ease and explain physicians' instructions. They must respect the confidential nature of medical information. Clinical duties require a reasonable level of manual dexterity and visual acuity.

Medical assistants may be able to advance to office manager. They may qualify for a variety of administrative support occupations or may teach medical assisting. With additional education, some enter other health occupations, such as nursing and medical technology.

Employment: Medical assistants held about 387,000 jobs in 2004. About 6 out of 10 worked in offices of physicians; about 14 percent worked in public and private hospitals, including inpatient and outpatient facilities; and 11 percent worked in offices of other health practitioners, such as chiropractors, optometrists and podiatrists. The rest worked mostly in outpatient care centres, public and private educational services, other ambulatory health care services, State and local government agencies, employment services, medical and diagnostic laboratories and nursing care facilities.

Job Outlook: Employment of medical assistants is expected to grow much faster than average for all occupations through the year 2014 as the health care industry expands because of technological advances in medicine and the growth and aging of the population. Increasing utilization of medical assistants in the rapidly growing health care industry will further stimulate job growth. In fact, medical assistants is projected to be one of the fastest growing occupations over the 2004–14 period.

Employment growth will be driven by the increase in the number of group practices, clinics and other health care facilities that need a high proportion of support personnel, particularly the flexible medical assistant who can handle both administrative and clinical duties. Medical assistants work primarily in outpatient settings, a rapidly growing sector of the health care industry.

In view of the preference of many health care employers for trained personnel, job prospects should be best for medical assistants with formal training or experience, particularly for those with certification.

Earnings: The earnings of medical assistants vary, depending on their experience, skill level and location. Median annual earnings of medical assistants were $24,610 in May 2004. The middle 50 percent earned between $20,650 and $28,930. The lowest 10 percent earned less than $18,010 and the highest 10 percent earned more than $34,650. Median annual earnings in the industries employing the largest numbers of medical assistants in May 2004 were:

Colleges, universities and professional schools	$27,490
Outpatient care centres	25,360
General medical and surgical hospitals	25,160
Offices of physicians	24,930
Offices of other health practitioners	21,930

Medical Records and Health Information Technicians

Significant Points: Employment is expected to grow much faster than average.

Job prospects should be very good; technicians with a strong background in medical coding will be in particularly high demand.

Entrants usually have an associate degree; courses include anatomy, physiology, medical terminology, statistics and computer science.

This is one of the few health occupations in which there is little or no direct contact with patients.

Nature of the Work: Every time a patient receives health care, a record is maintained of the observations, medical or surgical interventions and treatment outcomes. This record includes information that the patient provides concerning his or her symptoms and medical history, the results of examinations, reports of x rays and laboratory tests, diagnoses and treatment plans. Medical records and health information technicians organize and evaluate these records for completeness and accuracy.

Technicians assemble patients' health information. They make sure that patients' initial medical charts are complete, that all forms are completed and properly identified and signed and that all necessary information is in the computer. They regularly communicate with physicians and other health care professionals to clarify diagnoses or to obtain additional information.

Some medical records and health information technicians specialize in coding patients' medical information for insurance purposes. Technicians who specialize in coding are called *health information coders, medical record coders, coder/abstractors,* or *coding specialists*. These technicians assign a code to each diagnosis and procedure.

They consult classification manuals and also rely on their knowledge of disease processes. Technicians then use computer software to assign the patient to one of several hundred "diagnosis-related groups," or DRGs. The DRG determines the amount for which the hospital will be reimbursed if the patient is covered by Medicare or other insurance programmes using the DRG system. In addition to the DRG system, coders use other coding systems, such as those geared toward ambulatory settings or long-term care.

Some technicians also use computer programmes to tabulate and analyze data to improve patient care, control costs, provide documentation for use in legal actions, respond to surveys, or use in research studies. For example, *cancer* (or tumor) *registrars* maintain facility, regional and national databases of cancer patients. Registrars review patient records and pathology reports, assign codes for the diagnosis and treatment of different cancers and selected benign tumours. Registrars conduct annual followups on all patients in the registry to track their treatment, survival and recovery.

Physicians and public health organizations then use this information to calculate survivor rates and success rates of various types of treatment, locate geographic areas with high incidences of certain cancers and identify potential participants for clinical drug trials. Cancer registry data also is used by public health officials to target areas for the allocation of resources to provide intervention and screening.

Medical records and health information technicians' duties vary with the size of the facility where they work. In large to medium-sized facilities, technicians might specialize in one aspect of health information or might supervise health information clerks and transcriptionists while a medical records and health information administrator manages the department. (See the statement on medical and health services managers elsewhere in the *Handbook.*) In small facilities, a credentialed medical records and health information technician sometimes manages the department.

Working Conditions: Medical records and health information technicians usually work a 40-hour week. Some overtime may be required. In hospitals—where health information departments often are open 24 hours a day, 7 days a week—technicians may work day, evening and night shifts.

Medical records and health information technicians work in pleasant and comfortable offices. This is one of the few health occupations in which there is little or no direct contact with patients. Because accuracy is essential in their jobs, technicians must pay close attention to detail. Technicians who work at computer monitors for prolonged periods must guard against eyestrain and muscle pain.

Training, Other Qualifications and Advancement: Medical records and health information technicians entering the field usually have an associate degree from a community or junior college. In addition to general education, coursework includes medical terminology, anatomy and physiology, legal aspects of health information, coding and abstraction of data, statistics, database management, quality improvement methods and computer science. Applicants can improve their chances of admission into a programme by taking biology, chemistry, health and computer science courses in high school.

Hospitals sometimes advance promising health information clerks to jobs as medical records and health information technicians, although this practice may be less common in the future. Advancement usually requires 2 to 4 years of job experience and completion of a hospital's in-house training programme.

Most employers prefer to hire Registered Health Information Technicians (RHIT), who must pass a written examination offered by the American Health Information Management Association (AHIMA). To take the examination, a person must graduate from a 2-year associate degree programme accredited by the Commission on Accreditation for Health Informatics and Information Management Education (CAHIIM). Technicians trained in non-CAHIIM-accredited programmes or trained on the job are not eligible to take the examination. In 2005, CAHIIM accredited 184 programmes for health information technicians.

Experienced medical records and health information technicians usually advance in one of two ways—by specializing or managing. Many senior technicians specialize in coding, particularly Medicare coding, or in cancer registry. Most coding and registry skills are learned on the job. Some schools offer certificates in coding as part of the associate degree programme for health information technicians, although there are no formal degree programmes in coding. For cancer registry, there were 11 formal 2-year certificate programmes in 2005 approved by the National Cancer Registrars Association (NCRA). Some schools and employers offer intensive 1- to 2-week training programmes in either coding or cancer registry. Once coders and registrars gain some on-the-job experience, many choose to become certified. Certifications in coding are available either from AHIMA or from the American Academy of Professional Coders. Certification in cancer registry is available from the NCRA.

In large medical records and health information departments, experienced technicians may advance to section supervisor, overseeing the work of the coding, correspondence, or discharge sections, for example. Senior technicians with RHIT credentials may become director or assistant director of a medical records and health information department in a small facility. However, in larger institutions, the director usually is an administrator with a bachelor's degree in medical records and health information administration.

Employment: Medical records and health information technicians held about 159,000 jobs in 2004. About 2 out of 5 jobs were in hospitals. The rest were mostly in offices of physicians, nursing care facilities, outpatient care centres and home health care services. Insurance firms that deal in health matters employ a small number of health information technicians to tabulate and analyze health information. Public health departments also hire technicians to supervise data collection from health care institutions and to assist in research.

Job Outlook: Job prospects should be very good. Employment of medical records and health information technicians is expected to grow much faster than average for all occupations through 2014 because of rapid growth in the number of medical tests, treatments and procedures that will be increasingly scrutinized by health insurance companies, regulators, courts and consumers. Also, technicians will be needed to enter patient information into computer databases to comply with Federal legislation mandating the use of electronic patient records.

Although employment growth in hospitals will not keep pace with growth in other health care industries, many new jobs will, nevertheless, be created. The majority of new jobs is expected in offices of physicians as a result of increasing demand for detailed records, especially in large group practices. Rapid growth also is expected in home health care services, outpatient care centres and nursing and residential care facilities. Additional job openings will result from the need to replace technicians who retire or leave the occupation permanently.

Technicians with a strong background in medical coding will be in particularly high demand. Changing government regulations and the growth of managed care have increased the amount of paperwork involved in filing insurance claims. Additionally, health care facilities are having difficulty attracting qualified workers, primarily because of the lack of both formal training programmes and sufficient resources to provide on-the-job training for coders. Job opportunities may be especially good for coders employed through temporary help agencies or by professional services firms.

Some cancer registrars may have difficulty finding open positions in their geographic area because of a limited number of registrars employed by health care facilities and low job turnover. However, when a position does become vacant, qualified cancer registrars have excellent prospects because of the limited number of trained registrars available for employment.

Earnings: Median annual earnings of medical records and health information technicians were $25,590 in 2004. The middle 50 percent earned between $20,650 and $32,990. The lowest 10 percent earned less than $17,720 and the highest 10 percent earned more than $41,760. Median annual earnings in the industries employing the largest numbers of medical records and health information technicians in 2004 were as follows:

General medical and surgical hospitals	$26,640
Nursing care facilities	26,330
Outpatient care centres	23,870
Offices of physicians	22,130

2

Career in Alternative Health Care

Alternative Medicine

Until recently, traditional medical systems were considered obscure, esoteric and shrouded in mysticism. But now the healing methods of the East are not only gaining acceptance not just as an alternative line of treatment, but are also being integrated into mainstream healthcare as complementary systems.

Ayurveda: Ayurveda, literally meaning the science of life, aims at healing the individual as a whole, instead of merely at the molecular level. This ancient healing system is based on the theory that everything is composed of panchamahabhutas, or the five basic elements (akaash, jal, vayu, agni, dharti). The main source of our knowledge of Ayurveda is the Atharva Veda, which dates back to around 1200 BC.

Siddha: The basic principles and doctrines of Siddha are similar to those of Ayurveda. The human body is considered a conglomeration of three humours, seven body tissues and waste products. Proper consistency of these constituents in the body ensures good health.

Unani: The Unani system of medicine originated in Greece during 460-377 BC and was brought to India by the Arabs and Persians. Unani medicine is based on the 'humoral theory' (relating to four bodily fluids) with each humour leading to a specific temperament in a human being. The Unani system makes use of plants, minerals and animal products as curative agents to re-establish the person's original humoral constitution.

Naturopathy: Popularly referred to as the drug-less treatment of diseases, Naturopathy is based on the practice of applying the simple laws of nature to cure diseases. It pays particular attention to balanced dietary and living habits, adopting purificatory measures and using natural techniques such as hydrotherapy, cold packs, mud packs, baths (water, oil & sun), massage, etc.

Yoga: Elements of yoga have been used in traditional Indian medicine for thousands of years, though yoga therapy in its present form is a mere 80 years old—created by the marriage of traditional yoga with modern medicine. Yogic therapy comprises a wide range of mind/body practices, ranging from postural and breathing exercises to deep relaxation and meditation for promoting positive health and well-being as well as helping particular medical conditions.

Homeopathy: Homeopathy lays emphasis on strengthening the immune system and curing like with like. Homeopathy today enjoys wide acceptability, both here and abroad, because of its holistic and intrinsic values, the low cost of medication coupled with ease of administration and absence of toxic side effects. An indication of its popularity lies in the fact that the best homeopathic medicines are manufactured by German and American companies. In India there are over 1.5 lakh qualified homeopaths.

Tibetan Medicine: This ancient system of medicine recognises three forms of energy in the body — flame, wind and bile. An imbalance of these energies in any organ leads to illness. Inherent in the medicinal tradition is the use of precious pills made of herbs and other natural substances and prescribed according to the calendar.

Reiki: Reiki practitioners believe that we are born with a certain level of energy, which gets depleted through our daily activities. If the energy is depleted at a rate faster than it can be replenished, it leads to ill health. Reiki attempts to increase the overall energy stores of the body by activating the seven chakras.

Chiropracty: Chiropracty is a 5000-year-old non-invasive, non-surgical approach for managing ortho-neuro-skeletal disorders, problems of the spine and other chronic disorders by restoring normal body function. Circumventing surgery (in most cases) cuts down recovery time and cost of treatment virtually by half. Chiropracty is quite popular in countries like USA, UK, Australia and Germany.

Employment Opportunities: The future of alternative medicine is bright. In a developing country like India, alternative therapeutic systems have a definite role to play in alleviating sickness—both chronic and acute. The cost-effectiveness, efficacy, low toxicity, ease of administration and relative safety (few adverse effects) renders them invaluable as viable alternatives to conventional medicine.

In fact, WHO has assessed the total world market for alternative medicine at a whopping Rs. 51,210 crore. The market for herbal remedies alone is pegged at $5 trillion with an annual growth of 11 per cent.

Home to over 15,000 medicinal plants and one of the 12 leading bio-diverse countries of the world, India is sitting on a veritable green mine. Awakening to this tremendous potential, the government has announced a separate national policy for the Indian Systems of Medicine & Homeopathy (ISM&H) to boost and promote indigenous medicine. Plans are also afoot to modernise the hospitals specialising in Indian Systems of Medicine (ISM).

However, the lack of formulation and standardisation is a major problem that plagues this fledgling industry. There are as many as 4,000 recorded Ayurvedic formulations, combining different herbs and metals. These need to be identified and analysed and put through a series of tests before they can be released in the market. Extensive R&D is under way in this field currently.

What it Takes?: Like other forms of medicine, the minimum qualification for most courses in traditional medicine is 10+2 with PCB (Physics, Chemistry & Biology). However, for Unani, Siddha and Tibetan medicine, arts and humanities students can also apply. Additionally, for pursuing a course in Ayurveda, you need to be well versed in Sanskrit/ Hindi, while for Unani, some knowledge of Arabic/ Urdu is a must. Similarly for studying the Siddha system, you need knowledge of Tamil.

What you'll Make?: Alternative systems of medicine are beginning to offer decent career opportunities—in research as well as in practise. But like any other profession, success depends on a multitude of factors and the job scenario when you graduate.

While private practice is a popular choice for those specialising in these systems, homeopathic and Ayurvedic practitioners, for instance, can also seek employment under the Central Government Health Scheme and in state government and municipal hospitals and dispensaries all over the country. Starting salaries are in the range of Rs 8,000 plus perks.

If you are hesitant to start off on your own, working with an established practitioner or clinic for a while would help you gain the necessary confidence.

Combining two or more of these complimentary systems can also add to your repertoire. But be prepared to face competition from other systems of medicine, particularly allopathic.

Drug and pharmaceutical companies and research institutions also hire consultants and research scientists to work in their respective fields. With several recognised institutions offering full-fledged courses of study, there is considerable opportunity in the teaching and academic sector as well.

Where to Study?: As in the case of allopathic medicine, full-fledged bachelors and master's degrees in traditional medicine (*e.g.*, BUMS for Unani, BAMS for Ayurveda and BHMS for Homeopathy) are offered at a large number of specialist medical colleges all over the country.

In the 5-year BAMS course, you will not only study the allopathic system of medicine, but also traditional Indian Medicine, which includes Shalya Chikitsa (ENT), Shalya Chikitsa (surgery), Sukrita (gynaecology & obstetrics),

Panchkarma (purification therapy), etc. Similarly, for the other systems of medicine, discussed above.

As in the case of Allopathic medicine, you require Physics, Chemistry and Biology in Class 12 to be eligible for the courses. Selection is based on merit in the entrance exam.

Ayurveda:

- Bachelors in Ayurvedic Medicine & Surgery (BAMS) is a 51/2 -year course
- Bharati Vidyapeeth, Lal Bahadur Shastri Marg, Pune 411 030 (Deemed) (Mah)
- Gujarat Ayurved University, Admn. Bhavan, Hospital Road, Jamnagar 361008 (Guj)
- Jamia Hamdard, Hamdard Nagar, New Delhi 110 062 (UT)
- Rajeev Gandhi University of Health Sciences, 4th 'T' Block, Jayanagar, Bangalore 560 041 (Kar)
- University of Calicut, Calicut 673 635 (Ker)
- University of Delhi, Faculty of Ayurvedic & Unani Medicine, Delhi 11 0 007 (UT)
- University of Kerala, Thiruvananthapuram 695 034 (Ker)
- (For details and list of courses in Ayurveda.
- Homoeopathy
- BHMS (Bachelor of Homoeopathic Medicine & Surgery) — 5½-year course
- Guru Gobind Singh Indraparstha University, (Dr. B.R. Sur Homoeopathic College, Hospital & Research Centre, New Delhi 110028).
- Maharashtra University of Health Sciences, Nashik 422005
- North Gujarat University, University Road, Patan 384 265
- NTR University of Health Science, Hyderabad 500016 (AP)
- University of Calcutta, Kolkata 700073
- University of Delhi, (Nehru Homeopathy Medical College, New Delhi 110024

Naturopathy & Yogic Sciences: Accepting Yoga as a scientific tool for balanced and all-round development of the human personality, 32 Indian Universities have established Departments of Yoga to impart education ranging from Certificate, Diploma, Degree and Ph.D & Teacher's Training Programmes. However, presently, only five universities in India offer degree at their affiliated colleges.

Nutritionists

Nutritions and Dietics finds application in medicine, dentistry, veterinary sciences, agriculture and public health. The wide range of professionals and practitioners in all these fields need to know what can or cannot and what should or should not be in human and animal diet.

The study of nutrition implies an understanding of the components of the food we eat, studies the components which are essential, finds out what is harmful, determines the right amounts for consumption, studies the digestive process and the various reactions of these foodstuffs in the body. It addresses questions concerning healthy eating and increased productivity.

Dieticians deal with the practical means by which we can improve our general health and well being.

Significant Points: Most jobs are in hospitals, nursing care facilities and offices of physicians or other health practitioners.

Dietitians and nutritionists need at least a bachelor's degree in dietetics, foods and nutrition, food service systems management, or a related area.

Faster than average employment growth is expected; however, growth may be constrained if employers substitute other workers for dietitians and if limitations are placed on insurance reimbursement for dietetic services.

Those who have specialized training in renal or diabetic diets or have a master's degree should experience good employment opportunities.

Nature of the Work: Dietitians and nutritionists plan food and nutrition programmes and supervise the preparation and serving of meals. They help to prevent and treat illnesses by promoting healthy eating habits and recommending dietary modifications, such as the use of less salt for those with high blood pressure or the reduction of fat and sugar intake for those who are overweight.

Dietitians manage food service systems for institutions such as hospitals and schools, promote sound eating habits through education and conduct research. Major areas of practice include clinical, community, management and consultant dietetics.

Clinical dietitians provide nutritional services for patients in institutions such as hospitals and nursing care facilities. They assess patients' nutritional needs, develop and implement nutrition programmes and evaluate and report the results. They also confer with doctors and other health care professionals to coordinate medical and nutritional needs. Some clinical dietitians specialize in the management of overweight patients or in the care of critically ill or renal (kidney) and diabetic patients. In addition, clinical dietitians in nursing care facilities, small hospitals, or correctional facilities may manage the food service department.

Community dietitians counsel individuals and groups on nutritional practices designed to prevent disease and promote health. Working in places such as public health clinics, home health agencies and health maintenance organizations, community dietitians evaluate individual needs, develop nutritional care plans and instruct individuals and their families. Dietitians working in home health agencies provide instruction on grocery shopping and food preparation to the elderly, individuals with special needs and children.

Increased public interest in nutrition has led to job opportunities in food manufacturing, advertising and marketing. In these areas, dietitians analyze foods, prepare literature for distribution, or report on issues such as the nutritional content of recipes, dietary fiber, or vitamin supplements.

Management dietitians oversee large-scale meal planning and preparation in health care facilities, company cafeterias, prisons and schools. They hire, train and direct other dietitians and food service workers; budget for and purchase food, equipment and supplies; enforce sanitary and safety regulations; and prepare records and reports.

Consultant dietitians work under contract with health care facilities or in their own private practice. They perform nutrition screenings for their clients and offer advice on diet-related concerns such as weight loss and cholesterol reduction. Some work for wellness programmes, sports teams, supermarkets and other nutrition-related businesses. They may consult with food service managers, providing expertise in sanitation, safety procedures, menu development, budgeting and planning.

Working Conditions: Most full-time dietitians and nutritionists work a regular 40-hour week, although some work weekends. About 1 in 4 worked part time in 2004.

Dietitians and nutritionists usually work in clean, well-lighted and well-ventilated areas. However, some dietitians work in warm, congested kitchens. Many dietitians and nutritionists are on their feet for much of the workday.

Training, Other Qualifications and Advancement: High school students interested in becoming a dietitian or nutritionist should take courses in biology, chemistry, mathematics, health and communications. Dietitians and nutritionists need at least a bachelor's degree in dietetics, foods and nutrition, food service systems management, or a related area. College students in these majors take courses in foods, nutrition, institution management, chemistry, biochemistry, biology, microbiology and physiology. Other suggested courses include business, mathematics, statistics, computer science, psychology, sociology and economics.

Of the 46 States and jurisdictions with laws governing dietetics, 31 require licensure, 14 require certification and 1 requires registration. Requirements vary by State. As a result, interested candidates should determine the requirements of the State in which they want to work before sitting for any exam. Although not required, the Commission on Dietetic Registration of the American Dietetic Association (ADA) awards the Registered Dietitian credential to those who pass an exam after completing their academic coursework and supervised experience.

As of 2004, there were about 227 bachelor's and master's degree programmes approved by the ADA's Commission on Accreditation for Dietetics Education (CADE).

Supervised practice experience can be acquired in two ways. The first requires the completion of a CADE-accredited programme. As of 2004, there were more than 50 accredited programmes, which combined academic and supervised practice experience and generally lasted 4 to 5 years. The second option requires the completion of 900 hours of supervised practice experience in any of the 265 CADE-accredited internships. These internships may be full-time programmes lasting 6 to 12 months or part-time programmes lasting 2 years. To maintain a registered dietitian status, at least 75 credit hours in approved continuing education classes are required every 5 years.

Students interested in research, advanced clinical positions, or public health may need an advanced degree.

Experienced dietitians may advance to management positions, such as assistant director, associate director, or director of a dietetic department, or may become self-employed. Some dietitians specialize in areas such as renal, diabetic, cardiovascular, or pediatric dietetics. Others may leave the occupation to become sales representatives for equipment, pharmaceutical, or food manufacturers.

Employment: Dietitians and nutritionists held about 50,000 jobs in 2004. More than half of all jobs were in hospitals, nursing care facilities, outpatient care centres, or offices of physicians and other health practitioners. State and local government agencies provided about 1 job in 5—mostly in correctional facilities, health departments and other public-health-related areas.

Some dietitians and nutritionists were employed in special food services, an industry made up of firms providing food services on contract to facilities such as colleges and universities, airlines, correctional facilities and company cafeterias.

Other jobs were in public and private educational services, community care facilities for the elderly (which includes assisted-living facilities), individual and family services, home health care services and the Federal Government—mostly in the U.S. Department of Veterans Affairs.

Some dietitians were self-employed, working as consultants to facilities such as hospitals and nursing care facilities or providing dietary counselling to individuals.

Job Outlook: Employment of dietitians is expected to grow faster than the average for all occupations through 2014 as a result of increasing emphasis on disease prevention through improved dietary habits. A growing and aging population will boost the demand for meals and nutritional counselling in hospitals, residential care facilities, schools, prisons, community health programmes and home health care agencies. Public interest in nutrition and increased emphasis on health education and prudent lifestyles also will spur demand, especially in management. In addition to employment growth, job openings will result from the need to replace experienced workers who leave the occupation.

The number of dietitian positions in nursing care facilities and in State government hospitals is expected to decline, as these establishments continue to contract with outside agencies for food services. However, employment is expected to grow rapidly in contract providers of food services, in outpatient care centres and in offices of physicians and other health practitioners. With increased public awareness of obesity and diabetes, Medicare coverage may be expanded to include medical nutrition therapy for renal and diabetic patients. As a result, dietitians that have specialized training in renal or diabetic diets or have a master's degree should experience good employment opportunities.

Employment growth for dietitians and nutritionists may be constrained if some employers substitute other workers, such as health educators, food service managers and dietetic technicians. Growth also may be curbed by limitations on insurance reimbursement for dietetic services.

Earnings: Median annual earnings of dietitians and nutritionists were $43,630 in May 2004. The middle 50 percent earned between $35,940 and $53,370. The lowest 10 percent earned less than $27,500 and the highest 10 percent earned more than $63,760. In May 2004, median annual earnings in general medical and surgical hospitals, the industry employing the largest number of dietitians and nutritionists, were $44,050.

According to the American Dietetic Association, median annualized wages for registered dietitians in 2005 varied by practice area as follows: $53,800 in consultation and business; $60,000 in food and nutrition management; $60,200 in education and research; $48,800 in clinical nutrition/ambulatory care; $50,000 in clinical nutrition/long-term care; $44,800 in community nutrition; and $45,000 in clinical nutrition/acute care. Salaries also vary by years in practice, education level, geographic region and size of the community.

Speech Therapy and Audiology

The world of the hearing and speech impaired is a very different one. Speech therapists and audiologists help in bridging the gap between the fortunate and the less fortunate.

Where speech and language therapists assist people who have a speech or language disorder, audiologists deal with patients who have hearing problems. In recent years, the role of speech therapists and audiologists has received a lot of attention. These professionals, devoted to the diagnosis and treatment of hearing problems and speech impairments have been able to make a significant difference in the lives of people with speech and hearing defects.

Art Therapy

Art therapy programmes teach students how to use art to promote the physical, mental and emotional health of patients. Students learn drawing, painting and other forms of art. They also learn psychology and counselling techniques.

Most of us have had moments of frustration, perhaps so intense that we imagine banging our fists against the wall. (Or actually do it, ouch!) Often in times such as these people turn to therapists to help them understand their problems and learn to cope with life's stresses. An innovative form of psychotherapy is art therapy. Art therapy programmes use art and creativity to help patients express their emotions. For example, art therapists may ask patients to draw or paint a picture of what they're feeling. The belief behind art therapy is that the creative process is a healthy and productive way to resolve emotional conflicts.

In art therapy programmes, your course work focuses on both art and psychology. You take courses in psychopathology, mental illnesses and counselling techniques.

You also take art classes in several different mediums. This can include pottery, drawing and painting, to name a few. You then take courses that show how to combine evaluation, counselling and art to treat patients effectively. Overall, you become a skilled therapist as well as a skilled artist. This allows you to help patients grow creatively and emotionally.

With a degree in art therapy, you can work in private practice, hospitals, or nursing homes. You can also work for community, rehabilitation, or outpatient centres. Many art therapists work in prisons and schools.

Several four-year colleges and universities offer undergraduate programmes in art therapy. However, most people get a master's degree in art therapy after completing their bachelor's degree. About 25 schools offer master's degrees in art therapy. Typically they take two years to complete.

In addition, a few programmes offer doctoral degrees in art therapy. These usually take three to five years to complete after you finish your master's. Most people with doctorates become professors."

Fitness Career

The fitness mantra seems to be catching up as people are realizing the need to maintain good health with a regular fitness regimen. Aerobics, yoga, gyms and fitness therapy centres are coming up in large numbers to keep the body and mind in good shape. There are plenty of natural and non-invasive ways to tune up one's body and mind.

Fitness is not merely a sports man's pursuit. Younger people wish to chisel the body with appropriate exercise regimen. Senior citizens want to keep fit with walking exercises.

Expectant mothers exercise to complement their body rhythm. Cardiovascular ailments, blood pressure or diabetes—appropriate exercise can help with them all. Nowadays even a child is taught to shape up and shed excess fat if need be.

Till a decade ago, a *fitness career* was considered more as a hobby than as a profession. Today fitness is serious business and there are many opportunities in the fitness sector.

Fitness industry is booming with career opportunities.

- Fitness instructor
- Freelance fitness instructor
- Personal trainer
- Fitness coach
- Fitness consultant
- Fitness specialist
- Health and life style coordinator

Let us take a closer look at each one of the above listed career prospects in fitness industry:

Fitness Instructor: There is a resident fitness instructor in most gyms for teaching fitness exercises. Previously most of these instructors were self taught. With the increased sophistication in the fitness equipments and infrastructural facilities, gymnasiums are keen to employ only trained and educated fitness instructors. Some of the areas of specialized exercise are:

- High / low aerobics
- Step aerobics
- Kickboxing
- Strength training
- Yoga
- Pilates
- Water aerobics

The leisure industry has varied fitness job opportunities from entry level to management cadre. Fitness instructor's jobs in sports, spas, personal trainings are available in plenty. There are tremendous opportunities for such instructors in corporate environs where group fitness instructors are highly sought after.

Freelance Fitness Instructor: This is a more popular preference because there is flexibility for the fitness instructor. The income depends upon where the instructor works and how many classes he/she is able to take. The lessons can also be taught in person and followed up by telephone or e-mail. A freelance fitness instructor can also write books, articles, teach in seminar classes and workshops. He/she can also work with personal trainers, doctors, dieticians and other health, fitness and lifestyle professionals at a preferred pace.

Personal Trainer: A personal fitness trainer must have the right background, passion for work and discipline to stay in the profession. Most sportsperson are in need of personal trainers. The trainer should monitor the day-to-day improvements in fitness and should focus on continuous updating of his client with what is new.

Certification as a personal trainer is essential for this employment. A trainer must have a bachelors, Masters or doctoral degree in exercise science, kinesiology, exercise physiology, physical education or sports management. It is essential for the fitness trainer to provide motivation, professional expertise and personalized attention to the client. Qualified training certainly helps to assess the individual fitness levels.

A trainer should have basic knowledge of how the human anatomy works and how the body has to be maintained. A four to six year background in human anatomy, physiology, biomechanics and exercise prescription techniques is strongly advised. Credentials in nutrition are also recommended.

Fitness Coach: A fitness coach has a variety of specialized fitness options to choose from. Weight management, nutrition, stress reduction, health risk management, smoking cessation, control of conditions like blood pressure and diabetes—the field of training and management is wide. A fitness coach can make a difference to your health, body, mood, mind, energy levels and confidence.

Fitness Consultant: Fitness consultants are sought after by film stars, beauty queens, sports persons, industrialists and corporate heads. A fitness consultant must be proficient and trained in martial arts, sports and in exercise techniques and routines. The exercise regimen varies from person to person according to the specific personal requirements. A pregnant woman's concept of exercise is different from a cardiac patient from a person requiring cosmetic help.

Fitness consultants are in demand in fitness clubs where lot of energy, enthusiasm and 'can do' attitude to fitness is reflected. Fitness consultant is an exciting career with rewards to people who are committed and passionate about their work. Consultancy work can be done even for distance learning—online training programmes that are increasingly available in sports management, nutrition, personal fitness, sports therapies and aerobics.

Fitness Specialist: Fitness specialists help coach and instruct groups or individuals in activities such as aerobics, sports and exercise. The specialist plans, organizes, heads, instructs, directs fitness and wellness programmes. The specialist also demonstrates techniques and indulges in corrective measures to improve one's physical skills. The specialist should analyze, monitor client's physical condition and provide nutritional recommendations. Fitness specialists should also have the ability to provide first aid to injured persons, treat minor injuries and give massages and relief to soreness and strains.

Health and Life-style Coordinators: The scope of health and life style coordinators is increasing day by day with healthy eating and life style programmes becoming a rage with all age groups. Ability to implement and assist in coordination of health and wellness programmes is essential for a life style coordinator. A pro-active, well-organized approach with excellent communication and presentation skills are essential skills for a health coordinator. There are rewarding career opportunities and exciting challenges waiting in state-of-the-art work environments in corporate settings and fitness centres. A lifestyle coordinator should exhibit leadership qualities and ability to work in dynamic and competitive environment. There are tremendous career opportunities in media especially television.

Fitness Career Requirements

- A trainer should be highly professional. He/she should insist on the work-out right from the first meeting onwards.
- A trainer who does not train his/her own body lacks the dedication needed to inspire their clients.
- Reputed trainers shall abide by a code of ethics and professional standards.
- A trainer should not become commercial minded and start selling dietary supplements along with exercise regimen for his/her own benefit.
- A trainer should keep abreast of any advances and new developments in the field.
- A trainer should not be egoistical and dogmatic. He/she should be able to appreciate and accept the new methodologies in training and fitness that may be adopted elsewhere.

Fitness Career Prospects

The growth of fitness facilities and programmes, sophisticated exercise equipments with strong scientific foundations have resulted in additional job opportunities for exercise, sports and fitness professionals. People have begun to realize that the time and money spent on staying fit is well worth the pounds that are lost in the process.

Fitness careers offer excellent remuneration with additional attractive incentives like leave and compensatory benefits, pension and saving schemes and holiday offers. A qualified personal trainer charges anywhere from $ 50 to $ 100 for every single session of fitness training. Apart from the handsome returns that fitness careers offers, there is a personal satisfaction derived by helping the clients stay fit.

Fitness Training

Being fit has never been so popular, or as necessary as it is today. With millions of people eager to lose weight and get in shape, fitness training is one of the fastest growing careers in the health and fitness industry today. The demand for professionals like aerobics instructors, yoga instructors and personal and corporate trainers is catapulting upwards.

There was a time when the only people using personal trainers were professional athletes who needed help for injury management or excelling at their sport. Today people from all walks of life – from celebrities to senior citizens – are using personal trainers to help them learn how to exercise, lose weight, maintain all round fitness and adopt a healthier lifestyle.

The Work: As a fitness trainer you will train people in different aspects of physical fitness and help the obese and sedentary get into shape. You will instruct or coach groups or individuals in various exercise routines (weights, aerobics and flexibility training), besides monitoring their progress through methods such as BMI (body mass index) and cardiovascular levels. If required, you will also give them basic advice on health and nutrition. You will demonstrate the correct use of various training apparatus and gadgets such as trampolines, weights, rowing machines, etc.

Your professional training and experience will also equip you to design specific programmes for different people – keeping in mind their age, lifestyle and health parameters. Suggest forward-bending exercises to someone with a spinal problem and you'll only end up worsening the situation – making your poor client double up with pain!

Fitness trainers work in gyms, big hotels, health clubs, fitness centres, spas, tourist resorts and even cruiseliners. After gaining some experience you could choose to run your own fitness centre. Another lucrative option today is to organise workplace wellness and fitness programmes for large companies. Increasingly, companies are laying great emphasis on physical fitness over and above the fiscal fitness of the organisation. They are offering their employees the facility of a well-equipped company gym where as a fitness trainer you could be advising top-notch executives how to stay in good shape.

Because gyms and health clubs offer a whole variety of exercise routines such as weightlifting, aerobics, karate, kickboxing, spin cycling, yoga, pilates or tai chi, you can choose to specialise in the areas you are comfortable with.

Let's take a look at some of the different kinds of work you could be doing as part of the fitness industry:

Fitness trainers help clients assess their level of physical fitness and help them set and reach fitness goals. They also demonstrate various exercise routines and help clients improve their technique. They also keep records of their clients' exercise sessions to analyse their progress and physical fitness.

Personal trainers work with clients on a one-on-one basis with celebrities and others who like privacy while they work out—either at a gym or at the client's home. The work-out is specially tailored to suit the client's specific health and fitness requirements. Obviously, you would prescribe a far more exacting routine for a football player or swimmer as compared to that for a film star or company honcho.

Aerobics instructors conduct group work-out sessions that involve aerobics, stretching and muscle conditioning exercises. You could even conduct these classes in a gym or at your own studio.

Sports instructors coach professional and non-professional athletes on an individual basis. They organise, instruct, train and lead athletes specialising in indoor and outdoor sports or self-defence training such as judo and karate. Using their expertise in the sport, sports instructors evaluate the fitness level of the athlete and the athlete's opponents to devise a competitive game strategy.

Yoga and naturopathy experts work in yoga or fitness institutes and in hospitals as consultants or instructors. Similarly, you could also work as a personal trainer for the well-heeled client who does not have the time or desire to go to a public gym or for someone suffering from a specific health problem. As more and more people look for holistic alternative cures and remedies that are natural and free from side effects, naturopathy and yoga have great promise.

Employment Opportunities: Today, fitness in India is a whopping Rs.2,000 crore industry and most fitness centres are swanky studios offering an array of fitness regimes such as aerobics, kickboxing, yoga, dancercise and other wor-kouts with sophisticated machines. Moreover, be it at home or at the fitness centre having a qualified trainer has become the 'in-thing'.

With gyms and health clubs mushrooming all over the country, the demand for qualified instructors is going up sharply. And this spells good prospects for those aiming to pursue fitness as their career. Trainers with the 'right' qualification can teach just about anybody who can pay to be healthy and fit — from hard-working executives to the stressed-out CEOs, the politicians, the self-conscious student, the middle-aged housewife.

There are many factors driving the emergence of financial planners. For one, money decisions have become more

What it Takes?: Understandably, the first essential for this profession is an athletic body and loads of energy. Apart from a love for fitness, you need to practice what you preach. You can't possibly flaunt dark circles and a paunch, while exhorting your clients to pound the treadmill and do fifty push-ups! As a fitness instructor you will also need to keep abreast of the latest developments in health science.

Besides a good physique and determination to spend long hours in spandex, you must have good knowledge of human anatomy, diet, nutrition and other health and fitness related matters.

You also need to be innovative enough to vary the exercise routine to avoid monotony and boredom. Make sure you introduce an element of "fun", taking care to devise an upper and lower body work-out that exercises all muscle groups uniformly.

To learn the basics, you will need to enrol for a professional training programme. But treat the course as a mere kick-off point. Keep reading up on fitness and experiment continuously—there's no end to learning in this field as new research and equipment keeps hitting the headlines.

After finishing the course you can start with assisting a senior Aerobics Instructor before you start taking your own classes or become a personal instructor.

Good communication and interpersonal skills will hold you in good stead, as you have to deal with all kinds of people.

What you'll Make?: With the high premium placed on physical fitness and appearances, it pays to be fit... and help others become fit too!

While the pay may be a little low to start with, as you gain experience and develop a personal style and rapport your take-home dramatically improves. Of course the most lucrative jobs going are those of a personal trainer to the rich and famous and those with high-end fitness centres, spas and resorts.

Once you've acquired a reputation, you could also be conducting one of the numerous fitness programmes or health shows on popular TV channels. Besides boosting your popularity, it will also augment your clientele.

Where to Study?: You can go for a professional course like the Nike Aerobics Course or Reebok Instructor Certification programme or for any of the several reputed locally offered courses like those at Talwalkar's in Mumbai.

The basic course is for 80 hours, with around 30 hours of theory and the remaining made up of practical sessions. At the end of the course there are exams, both written and practical, to be passed before you can become a Reebok Certified Fitness Instructor. Except for Step Reebok, most programmes are not equipment-based.

In Delhi, Reebok India organises the course twice a year under the Reebok Instructor Alliance programme. The 2 ½-month 80-hour course culminates in an A-level Master Trainer Exam, which you must clear in order to be certified as trainer.

Only five colleges in India offer a Bachelor's Degree in Yoga & Naturopathy (5½ yrs). However, Central Council for Research in Yoga & Naturopathyhas formulated the syllabus for a 1-year Diploma in Yoga & Naturopathy (DYN) which is approved by the M/o Health & Family Welfare. The Council presently finances 17 centres for conducting these courses. There are numerous private centres as well. But you will need to ensure that they are not manned by self-taught quacks.

Similarly, if you wish to train in any of the martial arts (Judo, Kung Fu, Karate), please do so from a "belted" or certified trainer/expert. Acquiring skills in massage therapy, reflexology, accupressure will be an asset.

The Sports Authority of India (SAI) offers courses in Sports & Athletics Coaching in a large number of disciplines at its various branches.

- HVPM, Amravati 444605 (affiliated to Amravati Univ)
- Indira Gandhi Institute of Physical Education & Sports Sciences (IGIPESS) (affiliated to University of Delhi), B-Block, Vikaspuri, New Delhi 110018
- Lakshmibai National College of Physical Education, Kariavattom P.O., Trivandrum 695581
- Lakshmibai National Institute of Physical Education, Shaktinagar, Mela Road, Gwalior 474002
- SAI, Netaji Subhas National Institute of Sports, Patiala 147001
- SAI, NS Eastern Centre, Salt Lake City, Sector-III, Kolkata 700091
- SAI, NS South Centre, University Campus, Bangalore 560056

A number of institutes and universities impart sports education for coaches at the undergraduate and postgraduate level *i.e.* Bachelors in Physical Education (BPEd) and Masters in Physical Education (MPEd).

Fitness Workers

Significant Points: Many group fitness and personal training jobs are part time, but many workers increase their hours by working at several different facilities or at clients' homes.

Night and weekend working hours are common.

Most fitness workers need to be certified.

Employment prospects are expected to be good because of rapid growth in the fitness industry.

Nature of the Work: Fitness workers lead, instruct and motivate individuals or groups in exercise activities, including cardiovascular exercise, strength training and stretching. They work in commercial and nonprofit health clubs, country clubs, hospitals, universities, yoga and Pilates studios, resorts and clients' homes. Increasingly, fitness workers also are found in workplaces, where they organize and direct health and fitness programmes for employees of all ages.

Although gyms and health clubs offer a variety of exercise activities such as weightlifting, yoga, cardiovascular training and karate, fitness workers typically specialize in only a few areas.

Personal trainers work one-on-one with clients either in a gym or in the client's home. Trainers help clients assess their level of physical fitness and set and reach fitness goals. Trainers also demonstrate various exercises and help clients improve their exercise techniques. Trainers may keep records of their clients' exercise sessions to assess clients' progress toward physical fitness.

Group exercise instructors conduct group exercise sessions that involve aerobic exercise, stretching and muscle conditioning. Because cardiovascular conditioning classes often involve movement to music, outside of class instructors must choose and mix the music and choreograph a corresponding exercise sequence. Pilates and yoga are two increasingly popular conditioning methods taught in exercise classes. Instructors demonstrate the different moves and positions of the particular method; they also observe students and correct those who are doing the exercises improperly. Group exercise instructors are responsible for ensuring that their classes are motivating, safe and challenging, yet not too difficult for the participants.

Fitness directors oversee the fitness-related aspects of a health club or fitness centre. Their work involves creating and maintaining programmes that meet the needs of the club's members, including new member orientations, fitness assessments and work-out incentive programmes. They also select fitness equipment; coordinate personal training and group exercise programmes; hire, train and supervise fitness staff; and carry out administrative duties.

Fitness workers in smaller facilities with few employees may perform a variety of functions in addition to their fitness duties, such as tending the front desk, signing up new members, giving tours of the fitness centre, writing newsletter articles, creating posters and flyers and supervising the weight training and cardiovascular equipment areas. In larger commercial facilities, personal trainers are often required to sell their services to members and to make a specified number of sales. Some fitness workers may combine the duties of group exercise instructors and personal trainers and in smaller facilities, the fitness director may teach classes and do personal training.

Working Conditions: Most fitness workers spend their time indoors at fitness centres and health clubs. Fitness directors and supervisors, however, typically spend most of their time in an office, planning programmes and special events and tending to administrative issues. Those in smaller fitness centres may split their time among the office, personal training and teaching classes. Directors and supervisors generally engage in less physical activity than do lower-level fitness workers. Nevertheless, workers at all levels risk suffering injuries during physical activities.

Since most fitness centres are open long hours; fitness workers often work nights and weekends and even occasional holidays. Some may have to travel from place to place throughout the day, to different gyms or to clients' homes, to maintain a full work schedule.

Fitness workers generally enjoy a lot of autonomy. Group exercise instructors choreograph or plan their own classes and personal trainers have the freedom to design and implement their clients' work-out routines.

Training, Other Qualifications and Advancement: Personal trainers must obtain certification in the fitness field to gain employment, while group fitness instructors do not necessarily need certification to begin working.

The most important characteristic that an employer looks for in a new group fitness instructor is the ability to plan and lead a class that is motivating and safe. Group fitness instructors often get started by participating in exercise classes and some become familiar enough to successfully audition and begin teaching class. They also may improve their skills by taking training courses or attending fitness conventions. Most organizations encourage their group instructors to become certified and many require it.

In the fitness field, there are many organizations—some of which are listed in the last section of this statement—that offer certification. Becoming certified by one of the top certification organizations is increasingly important, especially for personal trainers. One way to ensure that a certifying organization is reputable is to see whether it is accredited or seeking accreditation by the National Commission for Certifying Agencies.

Most certifying organizations require candidates to have a high school diploma, be certified in cardiopulmonary resuscitation (CPR) and pass an exam. All certification exams have a written component and some also have a practical component. The exams measure knowledge of human physiology, proper exercise techniques, asscssment of client fitness levels and development of appropriate exercise programmes.

There is no particular training programme required for certifications; candidates may prepare however they prefer. Certifying organizations do offer study materials, including books, CD-ROMs, other audio and visual materials and exam preparation workshops and seminars, but exam candidates are not required to purchase materials to sit for the exams. Certification generally is good for 2 years, after which workers must become recertified by attending continuing education classes. Some organizations offer more advanced certification, requiring an associate or bachelor's degree in an exercise-related subject for individuals interested in training athletes, working with people who are injured or ill, or advising clients on whole-life health.

Training for Pilates and yoga teachers is changing. Because interest in these forms of exercise has exploded in recent years, the demand for teachers has grown faster than the ability to train them properly. However, because inexperienced teachers have contributed to student injuries, there has been a push toward more standardized, rigorous requirements for teacher training.

Pilates and yoga teachers usually do not need group exercise certifications like the ones described above. It is more important that they have specialized training in their particular method of exercise. For Pilates, training options range from weekend-long workshops to year-long programmes, but the trend is toward requiring more training.

The Pilates Method Alliance has established training standards that recommend at least 200 hours of training; the group also has standards for training schools and maintains a list of training schools that meet the requirements. However, some Pilates teachers are certified group exercise instructors who go through short Pilates workshops; currently, many fitness centres hire people with minimal Pilates training if the applicants have a fitness certification and group fitness experience.

Training requirements for yoga teachers are similar to those for Pilates teachers. Training programmes range from a few days to more than 2 years. Many people get their start by taking yoga; eventually, their teachers may consider them suited to assist or to substitute teach. Some students may begin teaching their own classes when their yoga teachers think they are ready; the teachers may even provide letters of recommendation.

Those who wish to pursue teaching more seriously usually then pursue formal teacher training. Currently, there are many training programmes through the yoga community as well as programmes through the fitness industry. The Yoga Alliance has established training standards of at least 200 training hours, with a specified number of hours in areas including techniques, teaching methodology, anatomy, physiology and philosophy. The Yoga Alliance also registers schools that train students to the standards. Because some schools may meet the standards but not be registered, prospective students should check the requirements and decide if particular schools meet them.

An increasing number of employers require fitness workers to have a bachelor's degree in a field related to health or fitness, such as exercise science or physical education. Some employers allow workers to substitute a college degree for certification, but most employers who require a bachelor's degree require both a degree and certification.

People planning fitness careers should be outgoing, good at motivating people and sensitive to the needs of others. Excellent health and physical fitness are important due to the physical nature of the job. Those who wish to be personal trainers in a large commercial fitness centre should have strong sales skills.

Fitness workers usually do not receive much on-the-job training; they are expected to know how to do their jobs when they are hired. The exception is newly certified personal trainers with no work experience, who sometimes begin by working alongside an experienced trainer before being allowed to train clients alone. Workers may receive some organizational training to learn about the operations of their new employer. They occasionally receive specialized training if they are expected to teach or lead a specific method of exercise or focus on a particular age or ability group.

A bachelor's degree and in some cases a master's degree, in exercise science, physical education, kinesiology, or a related area, along with experience, usually is required to advance to management positions in a health club or fitness centre. As in many fields, managerial skills are needed to advance to supervisory or managerial positions. College courses in management, business administration, accounting and personnel management may be helpful for advancement to supervisory or managerial jobs, but many fitness companies have corporate universities in which they train employees for management positions.

Personal trainers may advance to head trainer, with responsibility for hiring and overseeing the personal training staff and for bringing in new personal training clients. Group fitness instructors may be promoted to group exercise director, responsible for hiring instructors and coordinating exercise classes. A next possible step is the fitness director, who manages the fitness budget and staff. The general manager's main focus is on the financial aspect of the organization, particularly setting and achieving sales goals; in a small fitness centre, however, the general manager usually is involved with all aspects of running the facility.

Some workers go into business for themselves and open their own fitness centres.

Employment: Fitness workers held about 205,000 jobs in 2004. Almost all personal trainers and group exercise instructors worked in physical fitness facilities, health clubs and fitness centres, mainly in the amusement and recreation industry or in civic and social organizations. About 7 percent of fitness workers were self-employed; many of these were personal trainers, while others were group fitness instructors working on a contract basis with fitness centres. Many fitness jobs are part time and many workers hold multiple jobs, teaching and/or doing personal training at several different fitness centres and at clients' homes.

Job Outlook: Opportunities are expected to be good for fitness workers because of rapid growth in the fitness industry. Many job openings also will stem from the need to replace the large numbers of workers who leave these occupations each year.

Employment of fitness workers—who are concentrated in the rapidly growing arts, entertainment and recreation industry—is expected to increase much faster than the average for all occupations through 2014. An increasing number of people spend more time and money on fitness and more businesses are recognizing the benefits of health and fitness programmes and other services such as wellness programmes for their employees.

Aging baby boomers are concerned with staying healthy, physically fit and independent. They have become the largest demographic group of health club members. The reduction of physical education programmes in schools, combined with parents' growing concern about childhood obesity, has resulted in rapid increases in children's health club membership.

Increasingly, athletic youth also are hiring personal trainers and weight-training gyms for children younger than 18 are expected to continue to grow. Health club membership among young adults also has grown steadily, driven by concern with physical fitness and by rising incomes.

As health clubs strive to provide more personalized service to keep their members motivated, they will continue to offer personal training and a wide variety of group exercise classes. Participation in yoga and Pilates is expected to continue to grow, driven partly by the aging population demanding low-impact forms of exercise and relief from ailments such as arthritis.

Earnings: Median annual earnings of personal trainers and group exercise instructors in May 2004 were $25,470. The middle 50 percent earned between $17,380 and $40,030. The bottom 10 percent earned less than $14,530 while the top 10 percent earned $55,560 or more. Earnings of successful self-employed personal trainers can be much higher. Median annual earnings in the industries employing the largest numbers of fitness workers in May 2004 were as follows:

Other amusement and recreation industries	$28,670
Other schools and instruction	22,320
Civic and social organizations	20,530

Because many fitness workers work part time, they often do not receive benefits such as health insurance or retirement plans from their employers. They do get the unusual benefit of the use of fitness facilities at no cost.

Beauty Therapy

Today beauty care is a global multi-billion dollar industry that employs millions of people — from scientists and production engineers right up to your neighborhood pedicurist and mehndiwalli.

If you have an eye for beauty, enjoy interacting with people and delight in transforming a plain Jane into a stunning sophisticate, beautycare is a field you could excel in. Although tastes and trends keep changing, the basic job of beautycare professionals remains the same: to help people look their best!

The Work: As a Beautician you have a whole range of specialisations to choose from: beauty therapy, hair styling, make-up, massage, facials, manicure, pedicure, electrolysis, herbal beautycare, etc. There are other closely related jobs like those of a beauty lab assistant, health club instructor, cosmetic sales person, consultant, yoga and naturecure practioner, etc. While it is possible to practice more than one of these simultaneously, you can choose to specialise in any one—hair, skin or make-up—if that's where your interest lies.

If you are specialising in hair, the work would involve cutting, colouring and styling hair. To achieve professionalism and a good reputation you must blend your technical skills with a dash of creativity and imagination. Barbara, an expert hairdresser who runs her own South Delhi salon, says, "Shaping and styling hair gives me the greatest thrill... Making my clients look good gives me tremendous job satisfaction, besides the opportunity to expand my practise. Financially too, hairdressing is highly paying. Today I can afford all the luxuries of life."

The make-up artiste's job is to make the face look attractive by using complementary shades of colour to highlight the features while camouflaging and down-playing the flaws. It is fascinating to watch an expert create several faces on a single individual with a few deft strokes. This is a highly specialised field and a well paying one to boot. Besides bridal and party make-up, these make-up artistes are in great demand in the fashion, advertising, film, television and theatre industry. Screen make-up is a specialisation in itself.

The facial expert's main work is concerned with skin problems like acne, dark patches or premature wrinkles and providing appropriate facial treatment depending on the client's skin type and overall condition. An electrologist is a specialist trained in the permanent removal of superfluous hair and needs to be technically adept at handling the laser equipment.

A cosmetic salesperson requires excellent knowledge of grooming, skin, hair and nail care in addition to detailed knowledge of the products they promote across the counter. The ability to make each customer feel like a queen without being overly pushy is an art you must learn. With international cosmetic brands and perfumes, being increasingly marketed in the country, companies hire smart young women (and men) to man their counters at large departmental stores, shopping malls, duty-free shops and star-rated hotels.

Companies like Amway, Aviance, Avon, Oriflame recruit a large and growing network of women for direct selling of their line of popular cosmetics and beauty aids on a part-time basis. They conduct short orientation courses to familiarise you with their product line and sales techniques. Attractive commission on sales can fetch you a tidy extra income — without being tied down to a nine-to-five office routine.

Employment Opportunities: Thanks to the growing fashion, fitness and beauty consciousness coupled with rising incomes and beauty culture, cosmetology has emerged as a major occupational avenue with tremendous commercial potential. Spurred by new scientific developments, techniques, products and media hype, the Indian beauty industry has truly come of age, generating mega revenues.

In 2003, the cosmetic industry recorded a revenue of Rs.3000 crore while the skincare segment alone constituted Rs.1000 crore. The herbal segment, presently worth Rs.300 crore and growing at the rate of 40 per cent is perhaps the fastest growing.

With an average growth rate of 12 per cent, this industry is bound to generate a high employment potential along with the need for related services in the years ahead.

After gaining some hands-on experience, you could open your own beauty parlour or hairdressing salon or a combination of both and provide all beauty services — under one roof. To open your own parlour you need thorough professional knowledge of beauty culture, sufficient funds, an accessible location, quality equipment and materials and dollops of business sense.

What it Takes?: An interesting aspect of this field is that it does not demand high academic qualifications although a flair for the job is definitely an asset. Also the training period is generally brief and can even be taken up at a somewhat later stage in life. Even at the age of thirty or forty you can opt for a course in cosmetology or hairdressing or the myriad other specialisations—after the gates for most other career opportunities have closed.

Personal qualities include a pleasing, well-groomed personality, gentleness, dexterity, an eye for fashion, readyness to work with your hands, loads of stamina and a strong back (you may have to stand for long hours at a stretch), conversational ease and the knack of making your clients feel special and comfortable. You must create a soothing and relaxing atmosphere while maintaining high standards of efficiency, cleanliness and hygeine—nothing can be more off-putting to a client than a hurried, slap-dash or sloppy job. Also make sure you don't suffer from an allergic or asthmatic condition (the fumes, dyes and chemicals you'll inhale and handle could trigger off an attack).

What you'll Make?: Starting out as fresh trainee or understudy don't expect to be paid handsomely. Just concentrate on perfecting your skills and picking up the tricks of the trade. Be glad if you're paid Rs.3,000 or thereabouts to begin with. Once you've mastered the practical aspects of the job, clients will ask for you by name and that's when you can demand your price. Reasonably good hairdressers and make-up artistes earn upwards of Rs.25,000, tips extra. A make-up artiste charges anywhere from Rs.500 to Rs.4,000 to do a bridal or photographic make-up. Multiply that during the rushed wedding season– and you've made a tidy pile.

Where to Train?: There are countless courses on offer for fees ranging from Rs.5,000 to Rs.25,000. However, Don't go for fancy-sounding crash courses that drill a hole in your pocket and leave you none the wiser.

Training in cosmetology typically takes six to 12 months, with theory, demonstration and practicals being part of the course. Training is imparted by various vocational institutions like polytechnics as well as by reputed professionals in the field.

Nagpur University's BTech in Cosmetic Technology, perhaps the only one of its kind, enjoys a good reputation.

Where to Study?: There are countless courses on offer at fees ranging from Rs.5,000-40,000. However, don't go for fancy-sounding crash courses that drill a hole in your pocket and leave you none the wiser.

- Training in cosmetology typically takes 6-12 months comprising theory, demonstration and 'practicals'. Training is imparted by various vocational institutions like women's polytechnics as well as by reputed professionals in the field *e.g.* Shahnaz Hussain, Habib, Blossom Kochar, Bharti Taneja, Miriam Zaveri, Vandana Luthra, Ambika Pillai, etc.), many of whom operate through their franchisees in various cities. Check around in your city for similar privately run courses (VLCC, Berkowits, Alps, Biotique, Pivot Point, Shahnaz Herbal, Women's World, etc.) which enjoy good word-of-mouth reputation.
- Nagpur University offers a BTech in Cosmetic Technology, perhaps the only one of its kind.
- National & Regional Vocational Training Institutes for Women (M/o Labour, GoI) offer recognised courses in beautycare/cosmetology (Delhi, Noida, Allahabad, Bangalore, Mumbai, Kolkata, Vadodra, Hissar, Indore, Trivandrum, Tura). Some reputed cosmetic manufacturers also offer courses in various aspects of make-up and hairstyling from time to time, often inviting foreign experts to conduct the workshops.

- Pearl Academy of Fashion, A-21/13, Naraina Industrial Area, Phase II, New Delhi 110028 offers a Diploma in Fashion Media Make-up (1-yr).
- YWCA centres in major cities also offer courses in beautycare of a reasonable standard

Dietician

Do we eat to live or instead live to eat? GB Shaw seemed to have the answer when he said "there is no love sincerer than the love of food". Ironic in today's age of bumper harvests and overflowing granaries that lifestyle diseases and many health-related problems–obesity, blood pressure, heart and liver conditions–are brought on by eating wrong and eating too much.

As a Dietician you will assist infants, the elderly, the sick, the hospitalised, the obese, nursing mothers, sportspersons and a host of others either in a clinical setting (hospitals and nursing homes) or as a consultant in a speciality clinic, *e.g.*, for diabetics, kidney or coronary patients.

The Work: Many people confuse dieticians with nutritionists. Although both are aware of the nutritional values of foods besides supervising food preparation and its service, there is a difference. Dieticians guide the clueless on healthy eating habits and draw up a personalised food plan that meets the patient's dietary restrictions, occupational constraints, fitness and stress levels, etc. Other than planning meals, dieticians also look into the day-to-day functioning of the organisation.

The nutritionist, on the other hand, studies the effect of food (on humans) and the effect of heat, storage and other environmental factors on food (when it is cooked/served). The work mostly consists of preventing illnesses and rehabilitating patients after an illness (by planning for them their optimal dietary intake to hasten their recovery and educating them about what foods they should avoid).

What it Takes?: Besides the requisite academic qualifications, it helps to have a scientific temper. That you must have a genuine interest in helping people with health and nutrition goes without saying. Good communication skills are equally essential, as you'll have to convince and motivate your clients in simple layman's terms.

Majority of research on health and nutrition takes place in the West and accordingly they issue guidelines and lines of treatment. These would necessarily have to be 'Indianised' to suit our different body structure, climate and lifestyle. You must also be adaptable and willing to experiment with new approaches. A one-size-fits-all approach won't work in India where the gastronomic variety is matched only by the number of dialects we speak.

Employment Opportunities: If you enjoy working with people, you can plumb for a dietician's job in a hospital, nursing home or special clinic where you will chart out individual diet plans for the patients. You may also choose to work with large institutional canteens like those in defence establishments, educational institutions, residential schools, factories, call centres or old age homes to oversee the quality of the bulk-cooked meals. In health and fitness centres and spas you will treat obese clients or sports and fitness buffs and those with specific health problems. Star-rated hotels also have dieticians on their rolls to plan out meals for guests who have specific health problems in consultation with the chef.

You could even be working with NGOs and government agencies involved in educating specific segments of the population or in monitoring food and health programmes.

Research is yet another option you could consider. International organisations like the UN, UNICEF and WHO as well as those that come under the ministry of Human Resource Development and institutes such as the National Institute of Nutrition also employ these professionals.

Large packaged food manufacturers and food processing units also hire nutritionists and dieticians to advice them on development of new products.

If you have a flair for writing, you could take a journalistic spin-off by writing on health and nutrition and suggesting innovative recipes and useful dietary tips with a focus on healthy and balanced eating. Most newspapers and magazines have separate health and fitness sections, which are very popular with readers. Similarly, almost all TV channels run popular health and fitness programmes which feature knowledgeable and articulate experts to discuss health issues and answer viewers' queries.

After you gain sufficient work experience, you may even consider setting up your own practice or work as a consultant to hospitals, clinics, sports teams, etc.

What you'll Make?: In hospitals, trainees generally receive a starting salary of Rs.3,000-5,000 per month, which may go up (after three months of service) to about Rs.8,000. The money also depends on the organisation you are working for--it generally hovers in the range of Rs.12,000 per month! However if you've built yourself a reputation and decide to set up your own practise or start your own health food restaurant or sales outlet–you could be on your way to riches villa!!

Best & Worst Bits: Since no two human beings are alike, the dietician's job can be quite varied and interesting. So what if milk is a no-no for someone with lactose intolerance — what else can you substitute so that he doesn't feel deprived or malnourished? Or how can fat-free food be dressed up with condiments to make it easy on the eyes and the taste buds?

Hopefully the health and diet consciousness that you will acquire in the course of your training and practice will also rub-off on you, your family and friends. Professionally too it makes good sense to be practising what you prescribe!

On the flip side, the only factor that can be called a 'con', if at all, is the time it takes for results to start showing up. Although in some cases, *i.e.*, post or pre-surgical care or management of diabetics and renal failure, they can be pretty dramatic.

Also your work, particularly in a clinical setting, will involve a lot of cajoling and convincing. Customary eating habits acquired over a lifetime are hard to change. Careful monitoring is also required in handling the critically ill and those with complex problems.

Where to Study?: A number of universities offer a 3-yr BSc/BA in Nutrition/Dietetics. These subjects are also offered as a postgraduate specialisation both at the degree (Masters in Home Sc/Applied Nutrition) as well as postgraduate diploma level.

Nuclear Medicine Technologists

Significant Points: About 7 out of 10 work in hospitals.

Nuclear medicine technology programmes range in length from 1 to 4 years and lead to a certificate, an associate degree, or a bachelor's degree. Faster than average growth will arise from an increase in the number of middle-aged and elderly persons, who are the primary users of diagnostic procedures.

The number of job openings each year will be relatively low because the occupation is small; technologists who also are trained in other diagnostic methods, such as radiologic technology or diagnostic medical sonography, will have the best prospects.

Nature of the Work: Diagnostic imaging embraces several procedures that aid in diagnosing ailments, the most familiar being the x ray. Another increasingly common diagnostic imaging method, called magnetic resonance imaging (MRI), uses giant magnets and radio waves, rather than radiation, to create an image. In nuclear medicine, radionuclides—unstable atoms that emit radiation spontaneously—are used to diagnose and treat disease.

Radionuclides are purified and compounded to form radiopharmaceuticals. Nuclear medicine technologists administer radiopharmaceuticals to patients and then monitor the characteristics and functions of tissues or organs in which the drugs localize. Abnormal areas show higher-than-expected or lower-than-expected concentrations of radioactivity. Nuclear medicine differs from other diagnostic imaging technologies because it determines the presence of disease on the basis of biological changes rather than changes in organ structure.

Nuclear medicine technologists operate cameras that detect and map the radioactive drug in a patient's body to create diagnostic images. After explaining test procedures to patients, technologists prepare a dosage of the radiopharmaceutical and administer it by mouth, injection, inhalation, or other means. They position patients and start a gamma scintillation camera, or "scanner," which creates images of the distribution of a radiopharmaceutical as it localizes in and emits signals from, the patient's body. The images are produced on a computer screen or on film for a physician to interpret.

When preparing radiopharmaceuticals, technologists adhere to safety standards that keep the radiation dose to workers and patients as low as possible. Technologists keep patient records and record the amount and type of radionuclides that they receive, use and discard.

Radiologic technologists and technicians, diagnostic medical sonographers and cardiovascular technologists and technicians also operate diagnostic imaging equipment, but their equipment creates images by means of a different technology. Nuclear medicine technologists also perform radioimmunoassay studies that assess the behaviour of a radioactive substance inside the body. For example, technologists may add radioactive substances to blood or serum to determine levels of hormones or of therapeutic drugs in the body. Most nuclear medicine studies, such as cardiac function studies, are processed with the aid of a computer.

Working Conditions: Nuclear medicine technologists generally work a 40-hour week, perhaps including evening or weekend hours, in departments that operate on an extended schedule. Opportunities for part-time and shift work also are available. In addition, technologists in hospitals may have on-call duty on a rotational basis.

Physical stamina is important because technologists are on their feet much of the day and may lift or turn disabled patients.

Although the potential for radiation exposure exists in this field, it is kept to a minimum by the use of shielded syringes, gloves and other protective devices and by adherence to strict radiation safety guidelines. The amount of radiation in a nuclear medicine procedure is comparable to that received during a diagnostic x-ray procedure. Technologists also wear badges that measure radiation levels. Because of safety programmes, badge measurements rarely exceed established safety levels.

Training, Other Qualifications and Advancement: Many employers and an increasing number of States require certification or licensure. Aspiring nuclear medicine technologists should check the requirements of the State in which they plan to work. Certification is available from the American Registry of Radiologic Technologists and from the Nuclear Medicine Technology Certification Board. Some workers receive certification from both agencies. Nuclear medicine technologists must meet the minimum Federal standards on the administration of radioactive drugs and the operation of radiation detection equipment.

Nuclear medicine technology programmes range in length from 1 to 4 years and lead to a certificate, an associate degree, or a bachelor's degree. Generally, certificate programmes are offered in hospitals, associate degree programmes in community colleges and bachelor's degree programmes in 4-year colleges and universities. Courses cover the physical sciences, biological effects of radiation exposure, radiation protection and procedures, the use of radiopharmaceuticals, imaging techniques and computer applications.

One-year certificate programmes are for health professionals who already posses an associate degree—especially radiologic technologists and diagnostic medical sonographers—but who wish to specialize in nuclear medicine. The programmes also attract medical technologists, registered nurses and others who wish to change fields or specialize. Others interested in nuclear medicine technology have three options: a 2-year certificate programme, a 2-year associate degree programme, or a 4-year bachelor's degree programme.

The Joint Review Committee on Education Programmes in Nuclear Medicine Technology accredits most formal training programmes in nuclear medicine technology. In 2005, there were 100 accredited programmes in the continental United States and Puerto Rico.

Nuclear medicine technologists should be sensitive to patients' physical and psychological needs. They must pay attention to detail, follow instructions and work as part of a team. In addition, operating complicated equipment requires mechanical ability and manual dexterity.

Technologists may advance to supervisor, then to chief technologist and, finally, to department administrator or director. Some technologists specialize in a clinical area such as nuclear cardiology or computer analysis or leave patient care to take positions in research laboratories. Some become instructors in, or directors of, nuclear medicine technology programmes, a step that usually requires a bachelor's or master's degree in the subject. Others leave the occupation to work as sales or training representatives for medical equipment and radiopharmaceutical manufacturing firms or as radiation safety officers in regulatory agencies or hospitals.

Employment: Nuclear medicine technologists held about 18,000 jobs in 2004. About 7 out of 10 were in hospitals—private and government. Most of the rest were in offices of physicians or in medical and diagnostic laboratories, including diagnostic imaging centres.

Job Outlook: Employment of nuclear medicine technologists is expected to grow faster than the average for all occupations through the year 2014. Growth will arise from technological advancement, the development of new nuclear medicine treatments and an increase in the number of middle-aged and older persons, who are the primary users of diagnostic procedures, including nuclear medicine tests. However, the number of openings each year will be relatively low because the occupation is small. Technologists who also are trained in other diagnostic methods, such as radiologic technology or diagnostic medical sonography, will have the best prospects.

Technological innovations may increase the diagnostic uses of nuclear medicine. One example is the use of radiopharmaceuticals in combination with monoclonal antibodies to detect cancer at far earlier stages than is customary today and without resorting to surgery. Another is the use of radionuclides to examine the heart's ability to pump blood.

New nuclear medical imaging technologies, including positron emission tomography (PET) and single photon emission computed tomography (SPECT), are expected to be used increasingly and to contribute further to employment growth. The wider use of nuclear medical imaging to observe metabolic and biochemical changes during neurology, cardiology and oncology procedures also will spur demand for nuclear medicine technologists.

Nonetheless, cost considerations will affect the speed with which new applications of nuclear medicine grow. Some promising nuclear medicine procedures, such as positron emission tomography, are extremely costly and hospitals contemplating these procedures will have to consider equipment costs, reimbursement policies and the number of potential users.

Earnings: Median annual earnings of nuclear medicine technologists were $56,450 in May 2004. The middle 50 percent earned between $48,720 and $67,460. The lowest 10 percent earned less than $41,800 and the highest 10 percent earned more than $80,300. Median annual earnings of nuclear medicine technologists in May 2004 were $54,920 in general medical and surgical hospitals.

Radiation Therapists

Significant Points: Good job opportunities are expected; applicants who are certified and who possess a bachelor's or an associate degree or a certificate in radiation therapy should have the best prospects.

Employment is projected to grow faster than average.

Radiation therapists need good communication skills because their work involves a great deal of patient interaction.

Nature of the Work: Radiation therapy is the use of radiation to treat cancer in the human body. As part of a medical radiation oncology team, radiation therapists use machines—called linear accelerators—to administer radiation treatment to patients. Linear accelerators, used in a procedure called external beam therapy, project high-energy x-rays at targeted cancer cells. As the x-rays collide with human tissue, they produce highly energized ions that can shrink and eliminate cancerous tumours. Radiation therapy sometimes is used as the sole treatment for cancer, but usually is used in conjunction with chemotherapy or surgery.

The first step in the radiation treatment process is called simulation. During simulation, a radiation therapist uses an x-ray imaging machine to pinpoint the location of the tumor. The therapist also may use a computerized tomography or CT scan to help determine how best to direct the radiation to minimize damage to healthy tissue.

The therapist then positions the patient and adjusts the linear accelerator so that, during treatment, radiation exposure is concentrated on the tumor cells. The radiation therapist then develops a treatment plan in conjunction with a radiation oncologist (a physician who specializes in therapeutic radiology) and a dosimetrist (a technician who calculates the dose of radiation that will be used for treatment). The therapist later explains the treatment plan to the patient and answers any questions that the patient may have.

After simulation, the radiation therapist positions the patient and adjusts the linear accelerator to mirror the conditions that were established in simulation. Then the therapist leaves the room to administer the radiation treatment. From a separate room that is protected from the x-ray radiation, the therapist operates the linear accelerator and monitors the patient's condition through a TV monitor and an intercom system. Treatment can take anywhere from 10 to 30 minutes and is usually administered once a day, 5 days a week, for a period of 2 to 9 weeks.

During the treatment phase, the radiation therapist monitors the patient's physical condition to determine if any adverse side effects are taking place. In addition, the therapist must be aware of the patient's emotional condition. Because many patients are under stress and are emotionally fragile, it is important for the therapist to maintain a positive attitude and provide emotional support. Radiation therapists also must keep detailed records of their patients' treatments. These records include information such as the dose of radiation used for each treatment, the total amount of radiation used to date, the area treated and the patient's reactions. Radiation oncologists and dosimetrists review these records to ensure that the treatment plan is working, to monitor the amount of radiation exposure that the patient has received and to keep unwanted side effects to a minimum.

Radiation therapists also assist medical radiation physicists, who keep the linear accelerator working. Because radiation therapists often work alone during the treatment phase, they need to be able to check the linear accelerator for problems and make any adjustments that are needed. Therapists also may assist dosimetrists, who calculate the amount of radiation for each treatment. Therapists may perform the routine aspects of this process, called dosimetry, which involves complex mathematical computations.

Working Conditions: Radiation therapists work in hospitals or in cancer treatment centres. These places are clean, well lighted and well ventilated. Therapists do a considerable amount of lifting and must be able to help disabled patients get on and off treatment tables. Therapists also work on their feet most of the time. Therapists generally work 40 hours a week and, unlike other health care occupations, they normally work only during the day. However, because radiation therapy emergencies do occur, some therapists are required to be on call and may have to work outside of their normal hours.

Because they work around radioactive materials, radiation therapists take great care to ensure that they are not exposed to dangerous levels of radiation. Following standard safety procedures can prevent overexposure.

Training, Other Qualifications and Advancement: Employers generally require applicants to complete an associate or a bachelor's degree programme in radiation therapy. Individuals also may become qualified by completing an associate or a bachelor's degree programme in radiography, which is the study of radiological imaging and then completing a 12-month certificate programme in radiation therapy.

Radiation therapy programmes have core courses on radiation therapy procedures and the scientific theories behind these procedures. In addition, such programmes often include courses on human anatomy, human physiology, physics, algebra, precalculus, writing, public speaking, computer science and research methodology.

Some States require that radiation therapists be licensed by a State accrediting board. Some States, as well as many employers, also require that radiation therapists be certified by the American Registry of Radiologic Technologists (ARRT). In order to become ARRT-certified, an applicant needs to complete an accredited radiation therapy programme, adhere to ARRT ethical standards and pass the ARRT certification examination.

In 2005 there were 94 accredited radiation therapy programmes. While enrolled in an accredited radiation therapy programme, students who wish to become ARRT-certified must take classes that are related to the subject matter of the certification examination.

The certification examination covers radiation protection and quality assurance, clinical concepts in radiation oncology, treatment planning, treatment delivery and patient care and education. Candidates also must demonstrate competency in several clinical practices, which include patient care activities; simulation procedures; dosimetry calculations; fabrication of beam modification devices; low-volume, high-risk procedures; and radiation treatment procedures.

AART certification is valid for 1 year, after which therapists must renew their certification. Requirements for renewal include abiding by the ARRT ethical standards, paying the annual dues and satisfying the continuing education requirements. Continuing education requirements must be met every 2 years and include either the completion of 24 credits of radiation therapy-related courses or the successful attainment of ARRT certification in a discipline other than radiation therapy. Renewed certification, however, may not be required by all States or employers that require initial certification.

Individuals interested in becoming radiation therapists should be psychologically capable of working with cancer patients. They should be caring and empathetic because they work with patients who are ill and under stress. Individuals also need good communication skills because their work involves a great deal of patient interaction. They should be able to keep accurate, detailed records. They also should be physically fit because they work on their feet for long periods and lift and move disabled patients.

Experienced radiation therapists may advance to manage radiation therapy programmes in treatment centres or other health care facilities. Managers generally continue to treat patients while taking on management responsibilities. Other advancement opportunities include teaching, technical sales and research. With additional training and certification, therapists also can become dosimetrists, who use complex mathematical formulas to calculate proper radiation doses.

Employment: Radiation therapists held about 15,000 jobs in 2004. About 84 percent worked in the health care industry, primarily in hospitals and in physicians' offices. Another 13 percent worked for State and local governments.

Job Outlook: Good job opportunities are expected. Applicants who are certified and who possess a bachelor's or an associate degree or a certificate in radiation therapy should have the best prospects.

Employment of radiation therapists is projected to grow faster than average for all occupations during the 2004-14 period. As the U.S. population grows and ages, demand will increase for radiation treatment. As radiation technology advances, radiation treatment will be prescribed for an increasing proportion of cancer patients. In addition to new jobs created over the projection period, a number of job openings will result as experienced radiation therapists retire or leave the occupation for other reasons.

Earnings: The median annual earnings of radiation therapists in May 2004 were $57,700. The middle 50 percent earned between $47,380 and $69,650. The lowest 10 percent earned less than $38,550 and the highest 10 percent earned more than $83,340. Some employers also reimburse their employees for the cost of continuing education.

Occupational Therapist Assistants and Aides

Significant Points: Employment is projected to increase much faster than the average, reflecting growth in the number of individuals with disabilities or limited function who require therapeutic services.

Occupational therapist assistants generally must complete an associate degree or a certificate programme; in contrast, occupational therapist aides usually receive most of their training on the job.

In an effort to control rising health care costs, third-party payers are expected to encourage occupational therapists to delegate more hands-on therapy work to lower-paid occupational therapist assistants and aides.

Nature of the Work: Occupational therapist assistants and aides work under the direction of occupational therapists to provide rehabilitative services to persons with mental, physical, emotional, or developmental impairments. The ultimate goal is to improve clients' quality of life and ability to perform daily activities. For example, occupational therapist assistants help injured workers re-enter the labour force by teaching them how to compensate for lost motor skills or help individuals with learning disabilities increase their independence.

Occupational therapist assistants, commonly known as *occupational therapy assistants,* help clients with rehabilitative activities and exercises outlined in a treatment plan developed in collaboration with an occupational therapist. Activities range from teaching the proper method of moving from a bed into a wheelchair to the best way to stretch and limber the muscles of the hand. Assistants monitor an individual's activities to make sure that they are performed correctly and to provide encouragement. They also record their client's progress for the occupational therapist. If the treatment is not having the intended effect, or the client is not improving as expected, the therapist may alter the treatment programme in hopes of obtaining better results. In addition, occupational therapist assistants document the billing of the client's health insurance provider.

Occupational therapist aides typically prepare materials and assemble equipment used during treatment. They are responsible for a range of clerical tasks, including scheduling appointments, answering the telephone, restocking or ordering depleted supplies and filling out insurance forms or other paperwork. Aides are not licensed, so the law does not allow them to perform as wide a range of tasks as occupational therapist assistants.

Working Conditions: The hours and days that occupational therapist assistants and aides work vary with the facility and with whether they are full—or part-time employees. Many outpatient therapy offices and clinics have evening and weekend hours, to help coincide with patients' personal schedules.

Occupational therapist assistants and aides need to have a moderate degree of strength, because of the physical exertion required in assisting patients with their treatment. For example, assistants and aides may need to lift patients. Constant kneeling, stooping and standing for long periods also are part of the job.

Training, Other Qualifications and Advancement: An associate degree or a certificate from an accredited community college or technical school is generally required to qualify for occupational therapist assistant jobs. In contrast, occupational therapist aides usually receive most of their training on the job.

There were 135 accredited occupational therapist assistant programmes in 2005. The first year of study typically involves an introduction to health care, basic medical terminology, anatomy and physiology. In the second year, courses are more rigorous and usually include occupational therapist courses in areas such as mental health, adult physical disabilities, gerontology and pediatrics. Students also must complete 16 weeks of supervised fieldwork in a clinic or community setting. Applicants to occupational therapist assistant programmes can improve their chances of admission by taking high school courses in biology and health and by performing volunteer work in nursing care facilities, occupational or physical therapists' offices, or other health care settings.

Occupational therapist assistants are regulated in most States and must pass a national certification examination after they graduate. Those who pass the test are awarded the title "Certified Occupational Therapy Assistant."

Occupational therapist aides usually receive most of their training on the job. Qualified applicants must have a high school diploma, strong interpersonal skills and a desire to help people in need. Applicants may increase their chances of getting a job by volunteering their services, thus displaying initiative and aptitude to the employer.

Assistants and aides must be responsible, patient and willing to take directions and work as part of a team. Furthermore, they should be caring and want to help people who are not able to help themselves.

Employment: Occupational therapist assistants and aides held about 27,000 jobs in 2004. Occupational therapist assistants held about 21,000 jobs and occupational therapist aides held approximately 5,400. About 30 percent of jobs for assistants and aides were in hospitals, 23 percent were in offices of occupational therapists and 18 percent were in nursing care facilities. The rest were primarily in community care facilities for the elderly, home health care services, individual and family services and State government agencies.

Job Outlook: Employment of occupational therapist assistants and aides is expected to grow much faster than the average for all occupations through 2014. The impact of proposed Federal legislation imposing limits on reimbursement for therapy services may adversely affect the job market for occupational therapist assistants and aides in the short run. Over the long run, however, demand for occupational therapist assistants and aides will continue to rise because of the increasing number of individuals with disabilities or limited function. Job growth will result from an aging population, including the baby-boom generation, which will need more occupational therapy services. The increased prevalence of sensory disorders in children will increase the demand for occupational therapy services.

Increasing demand also will result from advances in medicine that allow more people with critical problems to survive and then need rehabilitative therapy. In an effort to control rising health care costs, third-party payers are expected to encourage occupational therapists to delegate more hands-on therapy work to lower-paid occupational therapist assistants and aides.

Earnings: Median annual earnings of occupational therapist assistants were $38,430 in May 2004. The middle 50 percent earned between $31,970 and $44,390. The lowest 10 percent earned less than $25,880 and the highest 10 percent earned more than $52,700. Median annual earnings of occupational therapist assistants were $40,130 in offices of other health practitioners, which includes offices of occupational therapists.

Median annual earnings of occupational therapist aides were $23,150 in May 2004. The middle 50 percent earned between $19,080 and $31,910. The lowest 10 percent earned less than $15,820 and the highest 10 percent earned more than $41,560.

Personal and Home Care Aides

Significant Points: Job opportunities are expected to be excellent because of rapid growth in home health care and high replacement needs.

Skill requirements are low, as is the pay.

About 33 percent of personal and home care aides work part time; most aides work with a number of different clients, each job lasting a few hours, days, or weeks.

Nature of the Work: Personal and home care aides help elderly, disabled, ill and mentally disabled persons live in their own homes or in residential care facilities instead of in health facilities. Most personal and home care aides work with elderly or physically or mentally disabled clients who need more extensive personal and home care than family or friends can provide.

Some aides work with families in which a parent is incapacitated and small children need care. Others help discharged hospital patients who have relatively short-term needs.

Personal and home care aides—also called *homemakers, caregivers, companions* and *personal attendants*—provide housekeeping and routine personal care services. They clean clients' houses, do laundry and change bed linens.

Aides may plan meals (including special diets), shop for food and cook. Aides also may help clients get out of bed, bathe, dress and groom. Some accompany clients to doctors' appointments or on other errands.

Personal and home care aides provide instruction and psychological support to their patients. They may advise families and patients on nutrition, cleanliness and household tasks. Aides also may assist in toilet training a severely mentally handicapped child, or they may just listen to clients talk about their problems.

In home health care agencies, a registered nurse, physical therapist, or social worker assigns specific duties and supervises personal and home care aides.

Aides keep records of services performed and of clients' condition and progress. They report changes in the client's condition to the supervisor or case manager. In carrying out their work, aides cooperate with health care professionals, including registered nurses, therapists and other medical staff.

Working Conditions: The personal and home care aide's daily routine may vary. Aides may go to the same home every day for months or even years. However, most aides work with a number of different clients, each job lasting a few hours, days, or weeks. Aides often visit four or five clients on the same day.

Surroundings differ from case to case. Some homes are neat and pleasant, whereas others are untidy and depressing.

Some clients are pleasant and cooperative; others are angry, abusive, depressed, or otherwise difficult.

Personal and home care aides generally work on their own, with periodic visits by their supervisor. They receive detailed instructions explaining when to visit clients and what services to perform for them. About one-third of aides work part time and some work weekends or evenings to suit the needs of their clients.

Aides are individually responsible for getting to the client's home. They may spend a good portion of the working day travelling from one client to another. Because mechanical lifting devices that are available in institutional settings are seldom available in patients' homes, aides must be careful to avoid overexertion or injury when they assist clients.

Training, Other Qualifications and Advancement: In some States, the only requirement for employment is on-the-job training, which generally is provided by most employers. Other States may require formal training, which is available from community colleges, vocational schools, elder care programmes and home health care agencies.

The National Association for Home Care and Hospice (NAHC) offers national certification for personal and home care aides. Certification is a voluntary demonstration that the individual has met industry standards. Certification requires the completion of a standard 75-hour course and written exam developed by NAHC. Home care aides seeking certification are evaluated on 17 different skills by a registered nurse.

Personal and home care aides should have a desire to help people and not mind hard work. They should be responsible, compassionate, emotionally stable and cheerful. In addition, aides should be tactful, honest and discreet because they work in private homes. Aides also must be in good health. A physical examination, including State-mandated tests such as those for tuberculosis, may be required. A criminal background check also may be required for employment. Additionally, personal and home care aides are responsible for their own transportation to reach patients' homes.

Advancement for personal and home care aides is limited. In some agencies, workers start out performing homemaker duties, such as cleaning. With experience and training, they may take on personal care duties. Some aides choose to receive additional training to become nursing and home health aides, licensed practical nurses, or registered nurses. Some experienced personal and home care aides may start their own home care agency.

Employment: Personal and home care aides held about 701,000 jobs in 2004. The majority of jobs were in home health care services; individual and family services; residential care facilities; and private households. Self-employed aides have no agency affiliation or supervision and accept clients, set fees and arrange work schedules on their own.

Job Outlook: Excellent job opportunities are expected for this occupation, because rapid employment growth and high replacement needs are projected to produce a large number of job openings.

Employment of personal and home care aides is projected to **grow much faster than average** for all occupations through the year 2014. The number of elderly people, an age group characterized by mounting health problems and requiring some assistance with daily activities, is projected to rise substantially. In addition to the elderly, other patients, such as the mentally disabled, will increasingly rely on home care. This trend reflects several developments, including efforts to contain costs by moving patients out of hospitals and nursing care facilities as quickly as possible; the realization that treatment can be more effective in familiar rather than clinical surroundings; and the development and improvement of medical technologies for in-home treatment.

In addition to job openings created by the increase in demand for these workers, replacement needs are expected to lead to many openings. The relatively low skill requirements, low pay and high emotional demands of the work result in high replacement needs. For these same reasons, many people are reluctant to seek jobs in the occupation. Therefore, persons who are interested in and suited for this work—particularly those with experience or training as personal care, home health, or nursing aides—should have excellent job prospects.

Earnings: Median hourly earnings of personal and home care aides were \$8.12 in May 2004. The middle 50 percent earned between \$6.83 and \$9.70 an hour. The lowest 10 percent earned less than \$5.93 and the highest 10 percent earned more than \$10.87 an hour. Median hourly earnings in the industries employing the largest numbers of personal and home care aides in May 2004 were as follows:

Residential mental retardation, mental health and substance abuse facilities	\$9.09
Vocational rehabilitation services	8.76
Community care facilities for the elderly	8.49
Individual and family services	8.48
Home health care services	6.99

Most employers give slight pay increases with experience and added responsibility. Aides usually are paid only for the time they work in the home, not for travel time between jobs. Employers often hire on-call hourly workers and provide no benefits.

Medical Transcriptionists

Significant Points: Job opportunities will be good.

Employers prefer medical transcriptionists who have completed a post-secondary training programme at a vocational school or community college.

Many medical transcriptionists telecommute from home-based offices as employees or subcontractors for hospitals and transcription services or as self-employed, independent contractors.

About 4 out of 10 worked in hospitals and another 3 out of 10 worked in offices of physicians.

Nature of the Work: Medical transcriptionists listen to dictated recordings made by physicians and other health care professionals and transcribe them into medical reports, correspondence and other administrative material. They generally listen to recordings on a headset, using a foot pedal to pause the recording when necessary and key the text into a personal computer or word processor, editing as necessary for grammar and clarity. The documents they produce include discharge summaries, history and physical examination reports, operative reports, consultation reports, autopsy reports, diagnostic imaging studies, progress notes and referral letters. Medical transcriptionists return transcribed documents to the physicians or other health care professionals who dictated them for review and signature, or correction. These documents eventually become part of patients' permanent files.

To understand and accurately transcribe dictated reports into a format that is clear and comprehensible for the reader, medical transcriptionists must understand medical terminology, anatomy and physiology, diagnostic procedures, pharmacology and treatment assessments. They also must be able to translate medical jargon and abbreviations into their expanded forms. To help identify terms appropriately, transcriptionists refer to standard medical reference materials—both printed and electronic; some of these are available over the Internet. Medical transcriptionists must comply with specific standards that apply to the style of medical records, in addition to the legal and ethical requirements involved with keeping patient information confidential.

Experienced transcriptionists spot mistakes or inconsistencies in a medical report and check to correct the information. Their ability to understand and correctly transcribe patient assessments and treatments reduces the chance of patients receiving ineffective or even harmful treatments and ensures high-quality patient care.

Currently, most health care providers transmit dictation to medical transcriptionists using either digital or analog dictating equipment. The Internet has grown to be a popular mode for transmitting documentation. Many transcriptionists receive dictation over the Internet and are able to quickly return transcribed documents to clients for approval. Another increasingly popular method utilizes speech recognition technology, which electronically translates sound into text and creates drafts of reports. Reports are then formatted; edited for mistakes in translation, punctuation, or grammar; and checked for consistency and any possible medical errors. Transcriptionists working in areas with standardized terminology, such as radiology or pathology, are more likely to encounter speech recognition technology.

However, use of speech recognition technology will become more widespread as the technology becomes more sophisticated.

Medical transcriptionists who work in physicians' offices may have other office duties, such as receiving patients, scheduling appointments, answering the telephone and handling incoming and outgoing mail. Medical secretaries, discussed in the statement on secretaries and administrative assistants, also may transcribe as part of their jobs.

Court reporters, have similar duties, but with a different focus. They take verbatim reports of speeches, conversations, legal proceedings, meetings and other events when written accounts of spoken words are necessary for correspondence, records, or legal proof.

Working Conditions: The majority of these workers are employed in comfortable settings, such as hospitals, physicians' offices, transcription service offices, clinics, laboratories, medical libraries, government medical facilities, or their own homes. Many medical transcriptionists telecommute from home-based offices as employees or subcontractors for hospitals and transcription services or as self-employed, independent contractors.

Work in this occupation presents hazards from sitting in the same position for long periods. Workers can suffer wrist, back, neck, or eye problems due to strain and risk repetitive motion injuries such as carpal tunnel syndrome. The constant pressure to be accurate and productive also can be stressful.

Many medical transcriptionists work a standard 40-hour week. Self-employed medical transcriptionists are more likely to work irregular hours—including part time, evenings, weekends, or on call at any time.

Training, Other Qualifications and Advancement: Employers prefer to hire transcriptionists who have completed post-secondary training in medical transcription, offered by many vocational schools, community colleges and distance-learning programmes. Completion of a 2-year associate degree or 1-year certificate programme—including coursework in anatomy, medical terminology, legal issues relating to health care documentation and English grammar and punctuation—is highly recommended, but not always required. Many of these programmes include supervised on-the-job experience. Some transcriptionists, especially those already familiar with medical terminology from previous experience as a nurse or medical secretary, become proficient through refresher courses and training.

The American Association for Medical Transcription (AAMT) awards the voluntary designation Certified Medical Transcriptionist (CMT), to those who earn a passing score on a certification examination. As in many other fields, certification is recognized as a sign of competence. Because medicine is constantly evolving, medical transcriptionists are encouraged to update their skills regularly. Every 3 years, CMTs must earn continuing education credits to be recertified.

In addition to understanding medical terminology, transcriptionists must have good English grammar and punctuation skills, as well as proficiency with personal computers and word processing software. Normal hearing acuity and good listening skills also are necessary. Employers require applicants to take pre-employment tests and usually prefer individuals with experience.

With experience, medical transcriptionists can advance to supervisory positions, home-based work, editing, consulting, or teaching. With additional education or training, some become medical records and health information technicians, medical coders, or medical records and health information administrators.

Employment: Medical transcriptionists held about 105,000 jobs in 2004. About 4 out of 10 worked in hospitals and another 3 out of 10 worked in offices of physicians. Others worked for business support services; medical and diagnostic laboratories; outpatient care centres; and offices of physical, occupational and speech therapists and audiologists.

Job Outlook: Job opportunities will be good. Employment of medical transcriptionists is projected to grow faster than average for all occupations through 2014. Demand for medical transcription services will be spurred by a growing and aging population.

Older age groups receive proportionately greater numbers of medical tests, treatments and procedures that require documentation. A high level of demand for transcription services also will be sustained by the continued need for electronic documentation that can easily be shared among providers, third-party payers, regulators, consumers and health information systems. Growing numbers of medical transcriptionists will be needed to amend patients' records, edit documents from speech recognition systems and identify discrepancies in medical reports.

Contracting out transcription work overseas and advancements in speech recognition technology are not expected to significantly reduce the need for well-trained medical transcriptionists. Outsourcing transcription work abroad—to countries such as India, Pakistan, Philippines and the Caribbean—has grown more popular as transmitting confidential health information over the Internet has become more secure; however, the demand for overseas transcription services is expected only to supplement the demand for well-trained domestic medical transcriptionists.

In addition, reports transcribed by overseas medical transcription services usually require editing for accuracy by domestic medical transcriptionists before they meet domestic quality standards. Speech-recognition technology allows physicians and other health professionals to dictate medical reports to a computer that immediately creates an electronic document.

In spite of the advances in this technology, the software has been slow to grasp and analyze the human voice and the English language and the medical vernacular with all its diversity. As a result, there will continue to be a need for skilled medical transcriptionists to identify and appropriately edit the inevitable errors created by speech recognition systems and to create a final document.

Hospitals will continue to employ a large percentage of medical transcriptionists, but job growth there will not be as fast as in other industries. An increasing demand for standardized records should result in rapid employment growth in physicians' offices, especially in large group practices.

Earnings: Medical transcriptionists had median hourly earnings of $13.64 in May 2004. The middle 50 percent earned between $11.50 and $16.32. The lowest 10 percent earned less than $9.67 and the highest 10 percent earned more than $19.11. Median hourly earnings in the industries employing the largest numbers of medical transcriptionists in May 2004 were:

General medical and surgical hospitals	$13.83
Offices of physicians	13.40
Business support services	13.40

Compensation methods for medical transcriptionists vary. Some are paid based on the number of hours they work or on the number of lines they transcribe. Others receive a base pay per hour with incentives for extra production. Employees of transcription services and independent contractors almost always receive production-based pay.

Independent contractors earn more than do transcriptionists who work for others, but independent contractors have higher expenses than their corporate counterparts, receive no benefits and may face higher risk of termination than do employed transcriptionists.

Speech-Language Pathologists

Significant Points: About half work in educational services and most others were employed by health care and social assistance facilities.

A master's degree in speech-language pathology is the standard credential required for licensing in most States.

Employment is expected to grow because the expanding population in older age groups is prone to medical conditions that result in speech, language and swallowing problems.

Excellent job opportunities are expected.

Nature of the Work: Speech-language pathologists, sometimes called *speech therapists*, assess, diagnose, treat and help to prevent speech, language, cognitive-communication, voice, swallowing, fluency and other related disorders.

Speech-language pathologists work with people who cannot produce speech sounds, or cannot produce them clearly; those with speech rhythm and fluency problems, such as stuttering; people with voice disorders, such as inappropriate pitch or harsh voice; those with problems understanding and producing language; those who wish to improve their communication skills by modifying an accent; and those with cognitive communication impairments, such as attention, memory and problem solving disorders. They also work with people who have swallowing difficulties.

Speech, language and swallowing difficulties can result from a variety of causes including stroke, brain injury or deterioration, developmental delays or disorders, learning disabilities, cerebral palsy, cleft palate, voice pathology, mental retardation, hearing loss, or emotional problems. Problems can be congenital, developmental, or acquired.

Speech-language pathologists use qualitative and quantitative assessment methods, including standardized tests, as well as special instruments, to analyze and diagnose the nature and extent of speech, language and swallowing impairments. Speech-language pathologists develop an individualized plan of care, tailored to each patient's needs. For individuals with little or no speech capability, speech-language pathologists may select augmentative or alternative communication methods, including automated devices and sign language and teach their use.

They teach these individuals how to make sounds, improve their voices, or increase their oral or written language skills to communicate more effectively. They also teach individuals how to strengthen muscles or use compensatory strategies to swallow without choking or inhaling food or liquid. Speech-language pathologists help patients develop, or recover, reliable communication and swallowing skills so patients can fulfil their educational, vocational and social roles.

Speech-language pathologists keep records on the initial evaluation, progress and discharge of clients. This helps pinpoint problems, tracks client progress and justifies the cost of treatment when applying for reimbursement. They counsel individuals and their families concerning communication disorders and how to cope with the stress and misunderstanding that often accompany them. They also work with family members to recognize and change behaviour patterns that impede communication and treatment and show them communication-enhancing techniques to use at home.

Most speech-language pathologists provide direct clinical services to individuals with communication or swallowing disorders. In medical facilities, they may perform their job in conjunction with physicians, social workers, psychologists and other therapists.

Speech-language pathologists in schools collaborate with teachers, special educators, interpreters, other school personnel and parents to develop and implement individual or group programmes, provide counselling and support classroom activities. Some speech-language pathologists conduct research on how people communicate. Others design and develop equipment or techniques for diagnosing and treating speech problems.

Working Conditions: Speech-language pathologists usually work at a desk or table in clean comfortable surroundings. In medical settings, they may work at the patient's bedside and assist in positioning the patient.

In school settings they may work with students in an office or classroom. Some deliver services in the client's home. While the job is not physically demanding, it requires attention to detail and intense concentration. The emotional needs of clients and their families may be demanding. Most full-time speech-language pathologists work 40 hours per week; about 1 in 5 work part time. Those who work on a contract basis may spend a substantial amount of time travelling between facilities.

Training, Other Qualifications and Advancement: In 2005, 47 States required speech-language pathologists to be licensed if they worked in a health care setting and all States required a master's degree or equivalent. A passing score on the national examination on speech-language pathology, offered through the Praxis Series of the Educational Testing Service, is needed as well.

Other requirements typically are 300 to 375 hours of supervised clinical experience and 9 months of postgraduate professional clinical experience. Forty-one States have continuing education requirements for licensure renewal. Medicaid, Medicare and private health insurers generally require a practitioner to be licensed to qualify for reimbursement.

Only 11 States require this same license to practice in the public schools. The other States issue a teaching license or certificate that typically requires a master's degree from an approved college or university. Some States will grant a temporary teaching license or certificate to bachelor's degree applicants, but a master's degree must be earned in 3 to 5 years. A few States grant a full teacher's certificate or license to bachelor's degree applicants.

In 2004, 239 colleges and universities offered graduate programmes in speech-language pathology that are accredited by the Council on Academic Accreditation in Audiology and Speech-Language Pathology. While graduation from an accredited programme is not always required to become a speech-language pathologist, it may be helpful in obtaining a license or may be required to obtain a license in some States. Courses cover the anatomy, physiology and the development of the areas of the body involved in speech, language and swallowing; the nature of disorders; acoustics; and psychological aspects of communication. Graduate students also learn to evaluate and treat speech, language and swallowing disorders and receive supervised clinical training in communication disorders.

Speech-language pathologists can acquire the Certificate of Clinical Competence in Speech-Language Pathology (CCC-SLP) offered by the American Speech-Language-Hearing Association. To earn a CCC, a person must have a graduate degree and 400 hours of supervised clinical experience, complete a 36-week postgraduate clinical fellowship and pass the Praxis Series examination in speech-language pathology administered by the Educational Testing Service (ETS).

Speech-language pathologists should be able to effectively communicate diagnostic test results, diagnoses and proposed treatment in a manner easily understood by their patients and their families. They must be able to approach problems objectively and be supportive. Because a patient's progress may be slow, patience, compassion and good listening skills are necessary.

As speech-language pathologists gain clinical experience and engage in continuing professional education, many develop expertise with certain populations, such as pre-schoolers and adolescents, or disorders, such as aphasia and learning disabilities. Some may obtain board recognition in a speciality area, such as child language, fluency, or feeding and swallowing. Experienced clinicians may become mentors or supervisors of other therapists or be promoted to administrative positions.

Employment: Speech-language pathologists held about 96,000 jobs in 2004. About half were employed in educational services, primarily in pre-schools and elementary and secondary schools. Others were employed in hospitals; offices of other health practitioners, including speech-language pathologists; nursing care facilities; home health care services; individual and family services; outpatient care centres; and child day care centres.

A few speech-language pathologists are self-employed in private practice. They contract to provide services in schools, offices of physicians, hospitals, or nursing care facilities, or work as consultants to industry.

Job Outlook: Employment of speech-language pathologists is expected to grow about as fast as the average for all occupations through the year 2014. As the members of the baby boom generation continue to age, the possibility of neurological disorders and associated speech, language and swallowing impairments increases.

Medical advances are also improving the survival rate of premature infants and trauma and stroke victims, who then need assessment and possible treatment. An increased emphasis also has been placed on early identification of speech and language problems in young children.

The combination of growth in the occupation and an expected increase in retirements over the coming years should create excellent job opportunities for speech-language pathologists. Opportunities should be particularly favourable for those with the ability to speak a second language, such as Spanish.

In health care facilities, restrictions on reimbursement for therapy services may limit the growth of speech-language pathologists in the near term. However, over the long run, the demand for therapists should continue to rise as growth in the number of individuals with disabilities or limited function spurs demand for therapy services.

Employment in educational services will increase along with growth in elementary and secondary school enrollments, including enrollment of special education students. Federal law guarantees special education and related services to all eligible children with disabilities. Greater awareness of the importance of early identification and diagnosis of speech and language disorders will also increase employment.

The number of speech-language pathologists in private practice will rise due to the increasing use of contract services by hospitals, schools and nursing care facilities.

Earnings: Median annual earnings of speech-language pathologists were $52,410 in May 2004. The middle 50 percent earned between $42,090 and $65,750. The lowest 10 percent earned less than $34,720 and the highest 10 percent earned more than $82,420. Median annual earnings in the industries employing the largest numbers of speech-language pathologists in May 2004 were:

Offices of other health practitioners	$57,240
General medical and surgical hospitals	55,900
Elementary and secondary schools	48,320

According to a 2003 survey by the American Speech-Language-Hearing Association, the median annual salary for full-time certified speech-language pathologists who worked on a calendar-year basis, generally 11 or 12 months annually, was $48,000. Certified speech-language pathologists who worked 25 or fewer hours per week had a median hourly salary of $40.00. Starting salaries for certified speech-language pathologists with one to three years of experience were $42,000 for those who worked on a calendar-year. According to a 2004 survey by the American Speech-Language-Hearing Association, the median annual salary for speech-language pathologists in schools was $50,000 for those employed on an academic year basis (usually 9 or 10 months).

Health and Ethical Issues

Use of Aromatics: In some cases, an excessive use of perfumes may cause allergic reactions of the skin (specifically, acetophenone is a well-known allergen present in many perfumes).

It is important to note that there is no benefit from creating a perfume exclusively from natural materials. There are several reasons for this:

- Many natural aroma materials are in fact inherently toxic and are either banned or restricted by IFRA. These naturals have been replaced by safer artificial or synthetic materials.
- Virtually no modern perfumes will perform successfully without one or more musk aromas. Musk was traditionally taken from the male musk deer *Moschus moschiferus*. This required the slaughter of the animal and in practice, musk hunters did not discriminate between male and female, old and young. They killed them all, only to obtain the musk pod which was solely produced by the young male deer and only when in season.

"Musk deer are protected under national legislation in many countries where they are found. The musk deer populations of Afghanistan, Bhutan, India, Nepal and Pakistan are included in Appendix I of CITES, the Convention on International Trade in Endangered Species of Wild Fauna and Flora. This means that these musk deer and their derivatives are banned from international commercial trade."

It is the policy of many perfume companies to use synthetic musk in place of natural musk for ethical reasons. Many synthetic musks are available and those used are all approved safe by IFRA.

- There are many new synthetic aromas that bear no olfactory relationship to any natural material and yet modern perfumery depends on these new odours for the infinite variety of perfumes available today. Many synthetics have very beautiful aromas not available in nature.
- Perfume composed only of expensive natural materials could be very expensive. Synthetic aromatics make possible perfumes at reasonable prices.
- In the distillation of natural essential oils any biocides (including pesticides, herbicides, or fungicides) that have been applied while the plant is growing may be concentrated into the essential oil making the oil toxic. Unless the essential oil is distilled from a certified organic origin, it may be dangerous.

Medical Photographer

Also known as: Photographer, Medical:

Medical photographers photograph patients, specimens, operations and so on, for medical records. They also prepare visual aids such as slides and videos, which can be used for teaching and research purposes.

Work Activities: Medical photographers work in hospitals, medical schools and research institutions. They work in clinical photography, which involves taking photographs of patients' conditions and injuries and in surgical photography, which requires them to record operations. Their photographs are used to help doctors diagnose conditions early and to aid researchers and those involved in training medical staff.

Medical photographers make their own photographs and other diagrams, artwork and X-rays into slides for use in tutorials and lectures. It is often the responsibility of the photographer to check that copyright laws are followed when reproducing original work.

Medical photographers use standard photographic equipment, usually a 35mm camera and flash gun (or digital equivalent), as well as sophisticated technical equipment. They may have to set up the equipment for an endoscopy, which involves attaching a tube with a light source to a camera body. The doctor then feeds it inside the patient so that shots of internal organs and joints can be taken. Infrared or ultraviolet radiation may be used to record images that the eye cannot normally see. Medical photographers should also understand video, cine photography and closed-circuit television techniques. As well as surgical and clinical work, they may take photographs for medical journals and books and of special events that happen within the hospital.

Personal Qualities and Skills: An interest in science and medicine is as important as an interest in photography. You must be able to work in distressing situations. For example, you may have to photograph a post-mortem or someone who has been disfigured. You must be able to communicate effectively with medical, nursing and research staff and other professionals working within the field of medicine. You will also work alongside medical artists and audiovisual technicians.

As a medical photographer, you will have to follow the same health and safety rules as other medical professionals when working in the operating theatre. In clinical photography you will often deal with people who feel embarrassed or upset, so a tactful and friendly manner is vital.

Pay and Opportunities: Pay rates for medical photographers vary depending on whether they are employed or self-employed. NHS employees are paid on a rising scale within defined pay bands, according to their skills and responsibilities. The pay rates given below are approximate.

Medical photographers will be on Band 5 of the NHS Agenda for Change pay scales. From 2005-2006 this scale ran from £19,730 to £24,803. Trainees would be on Band 4 £16,405—£19,730. Specialist medical photographers will be on Band 6, £22,886—£31,004.

Working hours can vary. Some photographers work regular office hours, usually over a 37-hour week, Monday to Friday. Those who work in hospitals may be required to work shifts, which may include early starts, late finishes and work at weekends and on public holidays.

Medical photographers can be based in departments of medical illustration in hospitals, in medical schools, in private medicine and in research establishments. There is a lot of competition for posts.

Vacancies in hospitals are advertised in the British Journal of Photography and on the website of the Institute of Medical Illustrators.

The following information is sourced from government statistics. The government's definition of types of job is slightly different to that used in this programme. For this type of job, the most relevant Government-defined occupation is 'Photographers and audiovisual equipment operators'.

In 2001 there were 3,000 people working as 'Photographers and audiovisual equipment operators' in Scotland. 14 in every 10,000 employees working in Scotland were employed as 'Photographers and audiovisual equipment operators'.

Entry Routes and Training: Trainee medical photographers study part-time for professional qualifications awarded by either the British Institute of Professional Photography (BIPP) or the Institute of Medical Illustrators (IMI).

To begin your training you will need a media qualification (in photography or video) at degree or Higher National Diploma level. As from June 2004, all entrants to the profession will require a degree, which may lead to these professional qualifications being replaced by the new postgraduate qualifications in Medical Illustration.

Once you have entered the profession you can join the Institute of Medical Illustrators as a student.

Physical Therapists

Significant Points: Employment is expected to increase much faster than the average, as growth in the number of individuals with disabilities or limited functioning spurs demand for therapy services.

Job opportunities should be particularly good in acute hospital, rehabilitation and orthopedic settings.

After graduating from an accredited physical therapist educational programme, therapists must pass a licensure exam before they can practice.

Nearly 6 out of 10 physical therapists work in hospitals or in offices of physical therapists.

Nature of the Work: Physical therapists provide services that help restore function, improve mobility, relieve pain and prevent or limit permanent physical disabilities of patients suffering from injuries or disease. They restore, maintain and promote overall fitness and health. Their patients include accident victims and individuals with disabling conditions such as low-back pain, arthritis, heart disease, fractures, head injuries and cerebral palsy.

Therapists examine patients' medical histories and then test and measure the patients' strength, range of motion, balance and coordination, posture, muscle performance, respiration and motor function. They also determine patients' ability to be independent and reintegrate into the community or workplace after injury or illness. Next, physical therapists develop plans describing a treatment strategy, its purpose and its anticipated outcome. Physical therapist assistants, under the direction and supervision of a physical therapist, may be involved in implementing treatment plans with patients. Physical therapist aides perform routine support tasks, as directed by the therapist.

Treatment often includes exercise for patients who have been immobilized and lack flexibility, strength, or endurance. Physical therapists encourage patients to use their own muscles to increase their flexibility and range of motion before finally advancing to other exercises that improve strength, balance, coordination and endurance. The goal is to improve how an individual functions at work and at home.

Physical therapists also use electrical stimulation, hot packs or cold compresses and ultrasound to relieve pain and reduce swelling. They may use traction or deep-tissue massage to relieve pain.

Therapists also teach patients to use assistive and adaptive devices, such as crutches, prostheses and wheelchairs. They also may show patients exercises to do at home to expedite their recovery.

As treatment continues, physical therapists document the patient's progress, conduct periodic examinations and modify treatments when necessary. Besides tracking the patient's progress, such documentation identifies areas requiring more or less attention.

Physical therapists often consult and practice with a variety of other professionals, such as physicians, dentists, nurses, educators, social workers, occupational therapists, speech-language pathologists and audiologists.

Some physical therapists treat a wide range of ailments; others specialize in areas such as pediatrics, geriatrics, orthopedics, sports medicine, neurology and cardiopulmonary physical therapy.

Working Conditions: Physical therapists practice in hospitals, clinics and private offices that have specially equipped facilities, or they treat patients in hospital rooms, homes, or schools.

In 2004, most full-time physical therapists worked a 40-hour week; some worked evenings and weekends to fit their patients' schedules. About 1 in 4 physical therapists worked part time. The job can be physically demanding because therapists often have to stoop, kneel, crouch, lift and stand for long periods. In addition, physical therapists move heavy equipment and lift patients or help them turn, stand, or walk.

Training, Other Qualifications and Advancement: All States require physical therapists to pass a licensure exam before they can practice, after graduating from an accredited physical therapist educational programme.

According to the American Physical Therapy Association, there were 205 accredited physical therapist programmes in 2004. Of the accredited programmes, 94 offered master's degrees and 111 offered doctoral degrees. All physical therapist programmes seeking accreditation are required to offer degrees at the master's degree level and above, in accordance with the Commission on Accreditation in Physical Therapy Education.

Physical therapist programmes start with basic science courses such as biology, chemistry and physics and then introduce specialized courses, including biomechanics, neuroanatomy, human growth and development, manifestations of disease, examination techniques and therapeutic procedures. Besides getting classroom and laboratory instruction, students receive supervised clinical experience. Among the courses that are useful when one applies to a physical therapist educational programme are anatomy, biology, chemistry, social science, mathematics and physics. Before granting admission, many professional education programmes require experience as a volunteer in a physical therapy department of a hospital or clinic. For high school students, volunteering with the school athletic trainer is a good way to gain experience.

Physical therapists should have strong interpersonal skills in order to be able to educate patients about their physical therapy treatments. Physical therapists also should be compassionate and possess a desire to help patients. Similar traits are needed to interact with the patient's family.

Physical therapists are expected to continue their professional development by participating in continuing education courses and workshops. In fact, a number of States require continuing education as a condition of maintaining licensure.

Employment: Physical therapists held about 155,000 jobs in 2004. The number of jobs is greater than the number of practicing physical therapists, because some physical therapists hold two or more jobs. For example, some may work in a private practice, but also work part time in another health care facility.

Nearly 6 out of 10 physical therapists worked in hospitals or in offices of physical therapists. Other jobs were in home health care services, nursing care facilities, outpatient care centres and offices of physicians.

Some physical therapists were self-employed in private practices, seeing individual patients and contracting to provide services in hospitals, rehabilitation centres, nursing care facilities, home health care agencies, adult day care programmes and schools. Physical therapists also teach in academic institutions and conduct research.

Job Outlook: Employment of physical therapists is expected to grow much faster than the average for all occupations through 2014. The impact of proposed Federal legislation imposing limits on reimbursement for therapy services may adversely affect the short-term job outlook for physical therapists. However, over the long run, the demand for physical therapists should continue to rise as growth in the number of individuals with disabilities or limited function spurs demand for therapy services.

Job opportunities should be particularly good in acute hospital, rehabilitation and orthopedic settings, because the elderly receive the most treatment in these settings. The growing elderly population is particularly vulnerable to chronic and debilitating conditions that require therapeutic services. Also, the baby-boom generation is entering the prime age for heart attacks and strokes, increasing the demand for cardiac and physical rehabilitation. Further, young people will need physical therapy as technological advances save the lives of a larger proportion of newborns with severe birth defects.

Future medical developments also should permit a higher percentage of trauma victims to survive, creating additional demand for rehabilitative care. In addition, growth may result from advances in medical technology that could permit the treatment of more disabling conditions.

Widespread interest in health promotion also should increase demand for physical therapy services. A growing number of employers are using physical therapists to evaluate worksites, develop exercise programmes and teach safe work habits to employees in the hope of reducing injuries in the workplace.

Earnings: Median annual earnings of physical therapists were $60,180 in May 2004. The middle 50 percent earned between $50,330 and $71,760. The lowest 10 percent earned less than $42,010 and the highest 10 percent earned more than $88,580. Median annual earnings in the industries employing the largest numbers of physical therapists in May 2004 were:

Home health care services	$64,650
Nursing care facilities	61,720
Offices of physicians	61,270
General medical and surgical hospitals	60,350
Offices of other health practitioners	60,130

Recreational Therapists

Significant Points: Overall employment of recreational therapists is expected to grow more slowly than the average for all occupations, but employment of therapists who work in community care facilities for the elderly and in residential mental retardation, mental health and substance abuse facilities should grow faster than the average.

Opportunities should be best for persons with a bachelor's degree in therapeutic recreation, or in recreation with a concentration in therapeutic recreation.

Recreational therapists should be comfortable working with persons who are ill or who have disabilities.

Nature of the Work: Recreational therapists, also referred to as *therapeutic recreation specialists*, provide treatment services and recreation activities to individuals with disabilities or illnesses. Using a variety of techniques, including arts and crafts, animals, sports, games, dance and movement, drama, music and community outings, therapists treat and maintain the physical, mental and emotional well-being of their clients. Therapists help individuals reduce depression, stress and anxiety; recover basic motor functioning and reasoning abilities; build confidence; and socialize effectively so that they can enjoy greater independence, as well as reduce or eliminate the effects of their illness or disability.

In addition, therapists help integrate people with disabilities into the community by teaching them how to use community resources and recreational activities. Recreational therapists should not be confused with recreation workers, who organize recreational activities primarily for enjoyment.

In acute health care settings, such as hospitals and rehabilitation centres, recreational therapists treat and rehabilitate individuals with specific health conditions, usually in conjunction or collaboration with physicians, nurses, psychologists, social workers and physical and occupational therapists. In long-term and residential care facilities, recreational therapists use leisure activities—especially structured group programmes—to improve and maintain their clients' general health and well-being. They also may provide interventions to prevent the client from suffering further medical problems and complications related to illnesses and disabilities.

Recreational therapists assess clients on the basis of information the therapists learn from standardized assessments, observations, medical records, the medical staff, the clients' families and the clients themselves. They then develop and carry out therapeutic interventions consistent with the clients' needs and interests.

For example, clients who are isolated from others or who have limited social skills may be encouraged to play games with others and right-handed persons with right-side paralysis may be instructed in how to adapt to using their unaffected left side to throw a ball or swing a racket. Recreational therapists may instruct patients in relaxation techniques to reduce stress and tension, stretching and limbering exercises, proper body mechanics for participation in recreational activities, pacing and energy conservation techniques and individual as well as team activities. In addition, therapists observe and document a patient's participation, reactions and progress.

Community-based recreational therapists may work in park and recreation departments, special-education programmes for school districts, or programmes for older adults and people with disabilities. Included in the last group are programmes and facilities such as assisted-living, adult day care and substance abuse rehabilitation centres. In these programmes, therapists use interventions to develop specific skills, while providing opportunities for exercise, mental stimulation, creativity and fun. Although most therapists are employed in other areas, those who work in schools help counsellors, teachers and parents address the special needs of students, including easing disabled students' transition into adult life.

Working Conditions: Recreational therapists provide services in special activity rooms, but also plan activities and prepare documentation in offices. When working with clients during community integration programmes, they may travel locally to instruct the clients regarding the accessibility of public transportation and other public areas, such as parks, playgrounds, swimming pools, restaurants and theaters.

Therapists often lift and carry equipment, as well as lead recreational activities. Recreational therapists generally work a 40-hour week that may include some evenings, weekends and holidays.

Training, Other Qualifications and Advancement: A bachelor's degree in therapeutic recreation, or in recreation with a concentration in therapeutic recreation, is the usual requirement for entry-level positions. Persons may qualify for para-professional positions with an associate degree in therapeutic recreation or a health care related field. An associate degree in recreational therapy; training in art, drama, or music therapy; or qualifying work experience may be sufficient for activity director positions in nursing homes.

Approximately 150 programmes prepare students to become recreational therapists. Most offer bachelor's degrees, although some also offer associate, master's, or doctoral degrees. Programmes include courses in assessment, treatment and programme planning, intervention design and evaluation. Students also study human anatomy, physiology, abnormal psychology, medical and psychiatric terminology, characteristics of illnesses and disabilities, professional ethics and the use of assistive devices and technology.

Although certification is usually voluntary, most employers prefer to hire candidates who are certified therapeutic recreation specialists. The National Council for Therapeutic Recreation Certification is the certificatory agency. To become certified, specialists must have a bachelor's degree, pass a written certification examination and complete an internship of at least 480 hours. Additional requirements apply in order to maintain certification and to recertify. Some States require licensure or certification to practice recreational therapy.

Recreational therapists should be comfortable working with persons who are ill or who have disabilities. Therapists must be patient, tactful and persuasive when working with people who have a variety of special needs. Ingenuity, a sense of humour and imagination are needed to adapt activities to individual needs and good physical coordination is necessary to demonstrate or participate in recreational activities.

Therapists may advance to supervisory or administrative positions. Some teach, conduct research, or consult for health or social services agencies.

Employment: Recreational therapists held about 24,000 jobs in 2004. About 6 out of 10 were in nursing care facilities and hospitals. Others worked in State and local government agencies and in community care facilities for the elderly, including assisted-living facilities. The rest worked primarily in residential mental retardation, mental health and substance abuse facilities; individual and family services; Federal Government agencies; educational services; and outpatient care centres. Only a small number of therapists were self-employed, generally contracting with long-term care facilities or community agencies to develop and oversee programmes.

Job Outlook: Overall employment of recreational therapists is expected to grow more slowly than the average for all occupations through the year 2014. In nursing care facilities—the largest industry employing recreational therapists—employment will grow slightly faster than the occupation as a whole as the number of older adults continues to grow. Employment is expected to decline, however, in hospitals as services shift to outpatient settings and employers emphasize cost containment.

Fast employment growth is expected in the residential and outpatient settings that serve disabled persons, the elderly, or those diagnosed with mental retardation, mental illness, or substance abuse problems. Among these settings are community care facilities for the elderly (including assisted-living facilities); residential mental retardation, mental health and substance abuse facilities; and facilities that provide individual and family services (such as day care centres for disabled persons and the elderly). Opportunities should be best for persons with a bachelor's degree in therapeutic recreation or in recreation with an option in therapeutic recreation. Opportunities also should be good for therapists who hold specialized certifications, for example, in, aquatic therapy, meditation, or crisis intervention.

Health care facilities will support a growing number of jobs in adult day care and outpatient programmes offering short-term mental health and alcohol or drug abuse services. Rehabilitation, home health care and transitional programmes will provide additional jobs.

The rapidly growing number of older adults is expected to spur job growth for recreational therapy professionals and paraprofessionals in assisted-living facilities, adult day care programmes and other social assistance agencies. Continued growth also is expected in community residential care facilities, as well as in day care programmes for individuals with disabilities.

Earnings: Median annual earnings of recreational therapists were $32,900 in May 2004. The middle 50 percent earned between $25,520 and $42,130. The lowest 10 percent earned less than $20,130 and the highest 10 percent earned more than $51,800. In May 2004, median annual earnings for recreational therapists were $28,130 in nursing care facilities.

Recreation Workers

Significant Points: Educational requirements for recreation workers range from a high school diploma to a graduate degree. Competition will remain keen for full-time career positions in recreation. The recreation field offers an unusually large number of part-time and seasonal job opportunities.

Nature of the Work: People spend much of their leisure time participating in a wide variety of organized recreational activities, such as arts and crafts, the performing arts, camping and sports. Recreation workers plan, organize and direct these activities in local playgrounds and recreation areas, parks, community centres, religious organizations, camps, theme parks and tourist attractions. Increasingly, recreation workers also are being found in workplaces, where they organize and direct leisure activities for employees.

Recreation workers hold a variety of positions at different levels of responsibility. *Recreation leaders*, who are responsible for a recreation program's daily operation, primarily organize and direct participants. They may lead and give instruction in dance, drama, crafts, games and sports; schedule the use of facilities; keep records of equipment use; and ensure that recreation facilities and equipment are used properly.

Workers who provide instruction and coach groups in specialities such as art, music, drama, swimming, or tennis may be called *activity specialists*. *Recreation supervisors* oversee recreation leaders and plan, organize and manage recreational activities to meet the needs of a variety of populations. These workers often serve as liaisons between the director of the park or recreation centre and the recreation leaders.

Recreation supervisors with more specialized responsibilities also may direct special activities or events or oversee a major activity, such as aquatics, gymnastics, or performing arts. *Directors of recreation and parks* develop and manage comprehensive recreation programmes in parks, playgrounds and other settings. Directors usually serve as technical advisors to State and local recreation and park commissions and may be responsible for recreation and park budgets. (Workers in a related occupation, *recreational therapists,* help individuals to recover from or adjust to illness, disability, or specific social problems.

Camp counsellors lead and instruct children and teenagers in outdoor-oriented forms of recreation, such as swimming, hiking, horseback riding and camping. In addition, counsellors provide campers with specialized instruction in subjects such as archery, boating, music, drama, gymnastics, tennis and computers.

In resident camps, counsellors also provide guidance and supervise daily living and general socialization. *Camp directors* typically supervise camp counsellors, plan camp activities or programmes and perform the various administrative functions of a camp.

Working Conditions: Recreation workers may work in a variety of settings—for example, a cruise ship, a woodland recreational park, a summer camp, or a playground in the centre of a large urban community. Regardless of the setting, most recreation workers spend much of their time outdoors and may work in a variety of weather conditions. Recreation directors and supervisors, however, typically spend most of their time in an office, planning programmes and special events. Directors and supervisors generally engage in less physical activity than do lower level recreation workers. Nevertheless, recreation workers at all levels risk suffering injuries during physical activities.

Many recreation workers work about 40 hours a week. People entering this field, especially camp counsellors, should expect some night and weekend work and irregular hours. Many recreation jobs are seasonal.

Training, Other Qualifications and Advancement: Educational requirements for recreation workers range from a high school diploma—or sometimes less for those seeking many summer jobs—to graduate degrees for some administrative positions in large public recreation systems. Full-time career professional positions usually require a college degree with a major in parks and recreation or leisure studies, but a bachelor's degree in any liberal arts field may be sufficient for some jobs in the private sector.

In industrial recreation, or "employee services" as it is more commonly called, companies prefer to hire those with a bachelor's degree in recreation or leisure studies and a background in business administration.

Specialized training or experience in a particular field, such as art, music, drama, or athletics, is an asset for many jobs. Some jobs also require certification. For example, a lifesaving certificate is a prerequisite for teaching or coaching water-related activities. Graduates of associate's degree programmes in parks and recreation, social work and other human services disciplines also enter some career recreation positions. High school graduates occasionally enter career positions, but this is not common. Some college students work part time as recreation workers while earning degrees.

A bachelor's degree in a recreation-related discipline and experience are preferred for most recreation supervisor jobs and are required for higher level administrative jobs. However, an increasing number of recreation workers who aspire to administrative positions are obtaining master's degrees in parks and recreation, business administration, or public administration. Certification in the recreation field may be helpful for advancement. Also, many persons in other disciplines, including social work, forestry and resource management, pursue graduate degrees in recreation.

Programmes leading to an associate's or bachelor's degree in parks and recreation, leisure studies, or related fields are offered at several hundred colleges and universities. Many also offer master's or doctoral degrees in the field. In 2004, about 100 bachelor's degree programmes in parks and recreation were accredited by the National Recreation and Park Association (NRPA). Accredited programmes provide broad exposure to the history, theory and practice of park and recreation management. Courses offered include community organization; supervision and administration; recreational needs of special populations, such as the elderly or disabled; and supervised fieldwork. Students may specialize in areas such as therapeutic recreation, park management, outdoor recreation, industrial or commercial recreation, or camp management.

The NRPA certifies individuals for professional and technical jobs. Certified Park and Recreation Professionals must pass an exam; earn a bachelor's degree with a major in recreation, park resources, or leisure services from a programme accredited by the NRPA and the American Association for Leisure and Recreation; or earn a bachelor's degree and have at least 5 years of relevant full-time work experience. Continuing education is necessary to remain certified.

Persons planning recreation careers should be outgoing, good at motivating people and sensitive to the needs of others. Excellent health and physical fitness are often required, due to the physical nature of some jobs. Volunteer experience, part-time work during school, or a summer job can lead to a full-time career as a recreation worker. As in many fields, managerial skills are needed to advance to supervisory or managerial positions.

Employment: Recreation workers held about 310,000 jobs in 2004 and many additional workers held summer jobs in the occupation. Of those with year-round jobs as recreation workers, about 35 percent worked for local governments, primarily in park and recreation departments.

Around 11 percent of recreation workers were employed in civic and social organizations, such as the Boy Scouts or Girl Scouts or the Red Cross. Another 15 percent of recreation workers were employed by nursing and other personal care facilities.

The recreation field has an unusually large number of part-time, seasonal and volunteer jobs, including summer camp counsellors, craft specialists and after-school and weekend recreation programme leaders. In addition, many teachers and college students accept jobs as recreation workers when school is not in session. The vast majority of volunteers serve as activity leaders at local day camp programmes, or in youth organizations, camps, nursing homes, hospitals, senior centres and other settings.

Job Outlook: Competition will remain keen for career positions as recreation workers because the field attracts many applicants and because the number of career positions is limited compared with the number of lower level seasonal jobs. Opportunities for staff positions should be best for persons with formal training and experience gained in part-time or seasonal recreation jobs. Those with graduate degrees should have the best opportunities for supervisory or administrative positions. Job openings also will stem from the need to replace the large numbers of workers who leave the occupation each year.

Overall employment of recreation workers is expected to grow about as fast as the average for all occupations through 2014. People will spend more time and money on recreation, spurring growth in civic and social organizations and, to a lesser degree, State and local government. Much growth will be driven by retiring baby boomers, who, with more leisure time, high disposable income and concern for health and fitness, are expected to increase their consumption of recreation services. Job growth also will be driven by rapidly increasing employment in nursing and residential care facilities. Employment growth may be inhibited, however, by budget constraints that local governments may face over the 2004–14 projection period.

The large number of temporary, seasonal jobs in the recreation field typically are filled by high school or college students, generally do not have formal education requirements and are open to anyone with the desired personal qualities. Employers compete for a share of the vacationing student labour force and although salaries in recreation often are lower than those in other fields, the nature of the work and the opportunity to work outdoors are attractive to many.

Earnings: In May 2004, median annual earnings of recreation workers who worked full time were $19,320. The middle 50 percent earned between $15,640 and $25,380. The lowest paid 10 percent earned less than $13,260, while the highest paid 10 percent earned $34,280 or more. However, earnings of recreation directors and others in supervisory or managerial positions can be substantially higher. Most public and private recreation agencies provide full-time recreation workers with typical benefits; part-time workers receive few, if any, benefits. In May 2004, median annual earnings in the industries employing the largest numbers of recreation workers were as follows:

Nursing care facilities	$20,660
Local government	19,650
Individual and family services	19,260
Other amusement and recreation industries	17,060
Civic and social organizations	16,950

Respiratory Therapists

Significant Points: Job opportunities will be very good, especially for therapists with cardiopulmonary care skills or experience working with infants.

All States (except Alaska and Hawaii), the District of Columbia and Puerto Rico require respiratory therapists to obtain a license.

Hospitals will continue to employ the vast majority of respiratory therapists, but a growing number of therapists will work in other settings.

Nature of the Work: *Respiratory therapists* and *respiratory therapy technicians*—also known as respiratory care practitioners—evaluate, treat and care for patients with breathing or other cardiopulmonary disorders. Practicing under the direction of a physician, respiratory therapists assume primary responsibility for all respiratory care therapeutic treatments and diagnostic procedures, including the supervision of respiratory therapy technicians. Respiratory therapy technicians follow specific, well-defined respiratory care procedures under the direction of respiratory therapists and physicians. In clinical practice, many of the daily duties of therapists and technicians overlap; furthermore, the two have the same education and training requirements. However, therapists generally have greater responsibility than technicians. For example, respiratory therapists will consult with physicians and other health care staff to help develop and modify individual patient care plans.

Respiratory therapists also are more likely to provide complex therapy requiring considerable independent judgment, such as caring for patients on life support in intensive-care units of hospitals. In this statement, the term *respiratory therapists* includes both respiratory therapists and respiratory therapy technicians.

Respiratory therapists evaluate and treat all types of patients, ranging from premature infants whose lungs are not fully developed to elderly people whose lungs are diseased. Respiratory therapists provide temporary relief to patients with chronic asthma or emphysema, as well as emergency care to patients who are victims of a heart attack, stroke, drowning, or shock.

To evaluate patients, respiratory therapists interview them, perform limited physical examinations and conduct diagnostic tests. For example, respiratory therapists test patients' breathing capacity and determine the concentration of oxygen and other gases in patients' blood. They also measure patients' pH, which indicates the acidity or alkalinity of the blood. To evaluate a patient's lung capacity, respiratory therapists have the patient breathe into an instrument that measures the volume and flow of oxygen during inhalation and exhalation.

By comparing the reading with the norm for the patient's age, height, weight and sex, respiratory therapists can provide information that helps determine whether the patient has any lung deficiencies. To analyze oxygen, carbon dioxide and pH levels, therapists draw an arterial blood sample, place it in a blood gas analyzer and relay the results to a physician, who then may make treatment decisions.

To treat patients, respiratory therapists use oxygen or oxygen mixtures, chest physiotherapy and aerosol medications. When a patient has difficulty getting enough oxygen into his or her blood, therapists increase the patient's concentration of oxygen by placing an oxygen mask or nasal cannula on the patient and set the oxygen flow at the level prescribed by a physician. Therapists also connect patients who cannot breathe on their own to ventilators that deliver pressurized oxygen into the lungs. The therapists insert a tube into the patient's trachea, or windpipe; connect the tube to the ventilator; and set the rate, volume and oxygen concentration of the oxygen mixture entering the patient's lungs.

Therapists perform regular assessments of patients and equipment. If the patient appears to be having difficulty breathing or if the oxygen, carbon dioxide, or pH level of the blood is abnormal, therapists change the ventilator setting according to the doctor's orders or check the equipment for mechanical problems. In home care, therapists teach patients and their families to use ventilators and other life-support systems. In addition, therapists visit patients several times a month to inspect and clean equipment and to ensure its proper use. Therapists also make emergency visits if equipment problems arise.

Respiratory therapists perform chest physiotherapy on patients to remove mucus from their lungs and make it easier for them to breathe. For example, during surgery, anesthesia depresses respiration, so chest physiotherapy may be prescribed to help get the patient's lungs back to normal and to prevent congestion. Chest physiotherapy also helps patients suffering from lung diseases, such as cystic fibrosis, that cause mucus to collect in the lungs. Therapists place patients in positions that help drain mucus and then vibrate the patients' rib cages and instruct the patients to cough.

Respiratory therapists also administer aerosols—liquid medications suspended in a gas that forms a mist which is inhaled—and teach patients how to inhale the aerosol properly to ensure its effectiveness.

In some hospitals, therapists perform tasks that fall outside their traditional role. Therapists' tasks are expanding into areas such as pulmonary rehabilitation, smoking cessation counselling, disease prevention, case management and polysomnography—the diagnosis of breathing disorders during sleep, such as apnea. Respiratory therapists also increasingly treat critical care patients, either as part of surface and air transport teams or as part of rapid-response teams in hospitals.

Working Conditions: Respiratory therapists generally work between 35 and 40 hours a week. Because hospitals operate around the clock, therapists may work evenings, nights, or weekends. They spend long periods standing and walking between patients' rooms. In an emergency, therapists work under a great deal of stress. Respiratory therapists employed in home health care must travel frequently to the homes of patients.

Respiratory therapists are trained to work with hazardous gases stored under pressure. Adherence to safety precautions and regular maintenance and testing of equipment minimize the risk of injury. As in many other health occupations, respiratory therapists run the risk of catching an infectious disease, but carefully following proper procedures minimizes this risk.

Training, Other Qualifications and Advancement: Formal training is necessary for entry into this field. Training is offered at the post-secondary level by colleges and universities, medical schools, vocational-technical institutes and the Armed Forces. An associate's degree is required for entry into the field. Most programmes award associate's or bachelor's degrees and prepare graduates for jobs as advanced respiratory therapists. A limited number of associate's degree programmes lead to jobs as entry-level respiratory therapists. According to the Commission on Accreditation of Allied Health Education Programmes (CAAHEP), 51 entry-level and 329 advanced respiratory therapy programmes were accredited in the United States, including Puerto Rico, in 2005.

Among the areas of study in respiratory therapy are human anatomy and physiology, pathophysiology, chemistry, physics, microbiology, pharmacology and mathematics. Other courses deal with therapeutic and diagnostic procedures and tests, equipment, patient assessment, cardiopulmonary resuscitation, the application of clinical practice guidelines, patient care outside of hospitals, cardiac and pulmonary rehabilitation, respiratory health promotion and disease prevention and medical record-keeping and reimbursement.

The National Board for Respiratory Care (NBRC) offers certification and registration to graduates of programmes accredited by CAAHEP or the Committee on Accreditation for Respiratory Care (CoARC). Two credentials are awarded to respiratory therapists who satisfy the requirements: Registered Respiratory Therapist (RRT) and Certified Respiratory Therapist (CRT). Graduates from accredited entry-level or advanced-level programmes in respiratory therapy may take the CRT examination. CRTs who were graduated from advanced-level programmes and who meet additional experience requirements can take two separate examinations leading to the award of the RRT credential.

All States (except Alaska and Hawaii), the District of Columbia and Puerto Rico require respiratory therapists to obtain a license. Passing the CRT exam qualifies respiratory therapists for State licenses. Also, most employers require respiratory therapists to maintain a cardiopulmonary resuscitation (CPR) certification. Supervisory positions and intensive-care specialities usually require the RRT or at least RRT eligibility.

Therapists should be sensitive to patients' physical and psychological needs. Respiratory care practitioners must pay attention to detail, follow instructions and work as part of a team. In addition, operating advanced equipment requires proficiency with computers.

High school students interested in a career in respiratory care should take courses in health, biology, mathematics, chemistry and physics. Respiratory care involves basic mathematical problem solving and an understanding of chemical and physical principles. For example, respiratory care workers must be able to compute dosages of medication and calculate gas concentrations.

Respiratory therapists advance in clinical practice by moving from general care to the care of critically ill patients who have significant problems in other organ systems, such as the heart or kidneys. Respiratory therapists, especially those with bachelor's or master's degrees, also may advance to supervisory or managerial positions in a respiratory therapy department. Respiratory therapists in home health care and equipment rental firms may become branch managers. Some respiratory therapists advance by moving into teaching positions.

Employment: Respiratory therapists held about 118,000 jobs in 2004. More than 4 out of 5 jobs were in hospital departments of respiratory care, anesthesiology, or pulmonary medicine.

Most of the remaining jobs were in offices of physicians or other health practitioners, consumer-goods rental firms that supply respiratory equipment for home use, nursing care facilities and home health care services. Holding a second job is relatively common for respiratory therapists. About 13 percent held another job, compared with 5 percent of workers in all occupations.

Job Outlook: Job opportunities are expected to be very good, especially for respiratory therapists with cardiopulmonary care skills or experience working with infants. Employment of respiratory therapists is expected to increase faster than average for all occupations through the year 2014, because of substantial growth in the numbers of the middle-aged and elderly population—a development that will heighten the incidence of cardiopulmonary disease—and because of the expanding role of respiratory therapists in the early detection of pulmonary disorders, case management, disease prevention and emergency care.

Older Americans suffer most from respiratory ailments and cardiopulmonary diseases such as pneumonia, chronic bronchitis, emphysema and heart disease. As their numbers increase, the need for respiratory therapists will increase as well. In addition, advances in inhalable medications and in the treatment of lung transplant patients, heart attack and accident victims and premature infants (many of whom are dependent on a ventilator during part of their treatment) will increase the demand for the services of respiratory care practitioners.

Although hospitals will continue to employ the vast majority of therapists, a growing number can expect to work outside of hospitals in home health care services, offices of physicians or other health practitioners, or consumer-goods rental firms.

Earnings: Median annual earnings of respiratory therapists were $43,140 in May 2004. The middle 50 percent earned between $37,650 and $50,860. The lowest 10 percent earned less than $32,220 and the highest 10 percent earned more than $57,580. In general medical and surgical hospitals, median annual earnings of respiratory therapists were $43,140 in May 2004.

Median annual earnings of respiratory therapy technicians were $36,740 in May 2004. The middle 50 percent earned between $30,490 and $43,830. The lowest 10 percent earned less than $24,640 and the highest 10 percent earned more than $52,280. Median annual earnings of respiratory therapy technicians employed in general medical and surgical hospitals were $36,990 in May 2004.

Physical Therapist Assistants and Aides

Significant Points: Employment is projected to increase much faster than average; physical therapist aides may face keen competition from the large pool of qualified applicants.

Physical therapist assistants generally have an associate degree, but physical therapist aides usually learn skills on the job. About 60 percent of jobs are in hospitals or offices of physical therapists.

Nature of the Work: Physical therapist assistants and aides perform components of physical therapy procedures and related tasks selected by a supervising physical therapist. These workers assist physical therapists in providing services that help improve mobility, relieve pain and prevent or limit permanent physical disabilities of patients suffering from injuries or disease. Patients include accident victims and individuals with disabling conditions such as low-back pain, arthritis, heart disease, fractures, head injuries and cerebral palsy.

Physical therapist assistants perform a variety of tasks. Components of treatment procedures performed by these workers, under the direction and supervision of physical therapists, involve exercises, massages, electrical stimulation, paraffin baths, hot and cold packs, traction and ultrasound. Physical therapist assistants record the patient's responses to treatment and report the outcome of each treatment to the physical therapist.

Physical therapist aides help make therapy sessions productive, under the direct supervision of a physical therapist or physical therapist assistant. They usually are responsible for keeping the treatment area clean and organized and for preparing for each patient's therapy. When patients need assistance moving to or from a treatment area, aides push them in a wheelchair or provide them with a shoulder to lean on. Because they are not licensed, aides do not perform the clinical tasks of a physical therapist assistant.

The duties of aides include some clerical tasks, such as ordering depleted supplies, answering the phone and filling out insurance forms and other paperwork. The extent to which an aide or an assistant performs clerical tasks depends on the size and location of the facility.

Working Conditions: The hours and days that physical therapist assistants and aides work vary with the facility and with whether they are full—or part-time employees. Many outpatient physical therapy offices and clinics have evening and weekend hours, to help coincide with patients' personal schedules. About 30 percent of all physical therapist assistants and aides work part time.

Physical therapist assistants and aides need a moderate degree of strength because of the physical exertion required in assisting patients with their treatment. In some cases, assistants and aides need to lift patients. Constant kneeling, stooping and standing for long periods also are part of the job.

Training, Other Qualifications and Advancement: Physical therapist aides are trained on the job, but physical therapist assistants typically earn an associate degree from an accredited physical therapist assistant programme. Not all States require licensure or registration in order for the physical therapist assistant to practice. The States that require licensure stipulate specific educational and examination criteria. Complete information on practice acts and regulations can be obtained from the State licensing boards. Additional requirements may include certification in cardiopulmonary resuscitation (CPR) and other first aid and a minimum number of hours of clinical experience.

According to the American Physical Therapy Association, there were 238 accredited physical therapist assistant programmes in the United States as of 2004. Accredited physical therapist assistant programmes are designed to last 2 years, or 4 semesters and culminate in an associate degree. Programmes are divided into academic study and hands-on clinical experience.

Academic course work includes algebra, anatomy and physiology, biology, chemistry and psychology. Many programmes require that students complete a semester of anatomy and physiology and have certifications in CPR and other first aid even before they begin their clinical field experience. Both educators and prospective employers view clinical experience as integral to ensuring that students understand the responsibilities of a physical therapist assistant.

Employers typically require physical therapist aides to have a high school diploma, strong interpersonal skills and a desire to assist people in need. Most employers provide clinical on-the-job training.

Employment: Physical therapist assistants and aides held about 101,000 jobs in 2004. Physical therapist assistants held about 59,000 jobs, physical therapist aides approximately 43,000. Both work with physical therapists in a variety of settings. About 60 percent of jobs were in hospitals or in offices of physical therapists. Others worked primarily in nursing care facilities, offices of physicians, home health care services and outpatient care centres.

Job Outlook: Employment of physical therapist assistants and aides is expected to grow much faster than the average for all occupations through the year 2014. The impact of proposed

Federal legislation imposing limits on reimbursement for therapy services may adversely affect the short-term job outlook for physical therapist assistants and aides.

However, over the long run, demand for physical therapist assistants and aides will continue to rise, in accordance with the increasing number of individuals with disabilities or limited function. The growing elderly population is particularly vulnerable to chronic and debilitating conditions that require therapeutic services.

These patients often need additional assistance in their treatment, making the roles of assistants and aides vital. The large baby-boom generation is entering the prime age for heart attacks and strokes, further increasing the demand for cardiac and physical rehabilitation. In addition, future medical developments should permit an increased percentage of trauma victims to survive, creating added demand for therapy services.

Physical therapists are expected to increasingly utilize assistants to reduce the cost of physical therapy services. Once a patient is evaluated and a treatment plan is designed by the physical therapist, the physical therapist assistant can provide many aspects of treatment, as prescribed by the therapist.

Physical therapist assistants and aides with prior experience working in a physical therapy office or other health care setting will have the best job opportunities. Physical therapist aides may face keen competition from the large pool of qualified individuals with a high school diploma.

Earnings: Median annual earnings of physical therapist assistants were $37,890 in May 2004. The middle 50 percent earned between $31,060 and $44,050. The lowest 10 percent earned less than $24,110 and the highest 10 percent earned more than $52,110. Median annual earnings in the industries employing the largest numbers of physical therapists aides in May 2004 were:

Nursing care facilities	$40,360
General medical and surgical hospitals	37,790
Offices of other health practitioners	37,120

Median annual earnings of physical therapist aides were $21,380 in May 2004. The middle 50 percent earned between $17,990 and $26,310.

The lowest 10 percent earned less than $15,380 and the highest 10 percent earned more than $33,550. Median annual earnings of physical therapist aides in May 2004 were $21,120 in general medical and surgical hospitals and $20,360 in offices of physical therapists.

Bibliography

Albarran, Alan B. and Gregory G. Pitts: *The Radio Broadcasting Industry*, Boston, Allyn and Bacon, 2001.

Albrecht, Ulrich: *A Short Research Guide on Arms and Armed Forces*, New York, Facts on File, 1980.

Alexander, James: *Internships in Communications, Ames*, Iowa State University Press, 1995.

Allman, Paul: *Careers in Video and Digital Video*, New York: Rosen, 2001.

Anders, Peter: *Envisioning Cyberspace*, New York, McGraw-Hill, 1999.

Arkin, William M.: *Research Guide to Current Military and Strategic Affairs*, Washington, Institute for Policy Studies, 1981.

Baehr, H. and Gary A.: *Turning In On: A Reader in Women and Media*, London, Arnold, 1996.

Ball, Victoria Kloss: *Opportunities in Interior Design and Decorating Careers*, Chicago, VGM Career Horizons, 2002.

Barnouw, Erik: *A Tower in Babel: the History of Broadcasting in the United States to 1933*, New York, Oxford University Press, 1966.

Baucom, Alfred H.: *Hospitality Design for the Graying Generation: Meeting the Needs of a Growing Market*, New York, Wiley, 1996.

Baxter, John: *Australian Cinema*, Sydney, Pacific Books, 1970.

Beaman, Jim: *Interviewing for Radio*, New York, Routledge, 2000.

Berkowitz, Ira: *Vault Career Guide to Advertising*, New York, Vault, 2004.

Bertrand, Ina and Diane Collins: *Government and Film in Australia*, Sydney, Currency Press, 1981.

Bliss, Edward and James L. Hoyt: *Writing News for Broadcast*, New York, Columbia University Press, 1994.

Boella, Michael John: *Principles of Hospitality Law*, London, Cassell, 1999.

Bone, Jan, & Ana Fernandez: *Opportunities in Film Careers*, New York, VGM Career Books, 2004.

Bowers, C. A.: *The Cultural Dimension of Educational Computing: Understanding the Non-neutrality of Technology*, New York, Teachers' College Press; 1988.

Boyd, Andrew: *Broadcast Journalism: Techniques of Radio and TV News*, Woburn, Focal Press, 2001.

Brown, Douglas Robert: *The Restaurant Managers Handbook: How to Set Up, Operate, and Manage a Financially Successful Restaurant*. Lauderhill, Atlantic Pub., 1991.

Brown, James and Quaal Ward: *Radio-Television-Cable Management*, New York, McGraw Hill, 1998.

Bryant, Jennings: *Television and the American Family*, Hillsdale, Lawrence Erlbaum, 1990.

Buckingham, David: *Young People and the Media*, New York, Manchester University Press, 1993.

Buckner, Robert W.: *Site Selection: New Advancements in Methods and Technology*, New York, Lebhar-Friedman Books, 1998.

Caldwell, J. T.: *Electronic Media and Technoculture*, New Brusnwick, Rutgers University Press, 2000.

Careers in Focus: *Photography*, New York, Ferguson, 2004.

Carmouche, Rita: *Behavioural Studies in Hospitality Management*, New York, Chapman & Hall, 1995.

Carroll, Victoria: *Writing News for Television*, Ames, Iowa State University Press, 1997.

Cassiday, Doris, and Bruce Cassiday: *Careers in the Beauty Industry*, New York, Franklin Watts, 1978.

Clark, Mona: *Interpersonal Skills for Hospitality Managers*, London, Chapman Hill, 1995.

Clark, Roy Peter: *A Journalist Teaches Young Writers*, Portsmouth, Heinemann, 1987.

Cockburn, C. and Ormrod, S.: *Gender and Technology in the Making*, London, Sage, 1993.

Cohler, David Keith: *Broadcast Newswriting*, Englewood Cliffs, Prentice Hall, 1990.

Cracknell, H. L.: *Escoffier: The Complete Guide to the Art of Modern Cookery*, New York, John Wiley, 1979.

Craig, James: *Graphic Design Career Guide*, New York, Watson-Guptill, 1992.

Crawford, Tad: *Starting Your Career As a Freelance Photographer*, New York, Allworth Press, 2003.

Crouse, Chuck: *Reporting for Radio*, Chicago, Bonus Books, 1998.

Davidson, M. J. and Cooper, C. L.: *Women and Information Technology*, New York, John Wiley & Sons, 1987.

Delaney, Chuck: *Photography Your Way*, New York, Allworth Press, 2005.

Dennis, Everette E. and Edward C. Pease: *Children and the Media*, New Brunswick, Transaction Publishers, 1996.

Diamond, S. Taylor's Way: *Women, Cultures and Technology*, New York: Routledge; 1997.

Donald, Ralph and Thomas Spann: *Fundamentals of Television Production*, Ames, Iowa State University Press, 2000.

Dornenburg, Andrew: *Culinary Artistry*, New York, John Wiley & Sons, 1996.

Douglas, George H.: *The Early Days of Radio Broadcasting*, Jefferson, NC: McFarland, 1987.

Easlea, B.: *Fathering the Unthinkable: Masculinity, Scientists and the Nuclear Arms Race*, London, Pluto Press, 1982.

Ellis, Elmo: *Opportunities in Broadcasting Careers*, Chicago, VGM Career Books, 2005.

Faulkner, W. and Arnold, E.: *Smothered by Invention: Technology in Women's Lives*, London, Pluto Press, 1985.

Fensch, Thomas: *Television News Anchors*, Jefferson, McFarland, 1993.

Field, Shelly: *Career Opportunities in Advertising and Public Relations*, New York, Ferguson, 2006.

Foster, Timothy R. V.: *How to Succeed As an Independent Consultant*, London: Kogan, Page, 2002.

Fox Keller, E.: *Reflections on Gender and Science*, New Haven, Yale University Press, 1985.

Gardner, Garth: *Careers in Computer Graphics and Animation*, Fairfax, GGC, 2001.

Gibbs, Jenny: *Interior Design*, New York, H. N. Abrams, 2005.

Go, Frank M.: *Human Resource Management in the Hospitality Industry*, New York, Wiley, 1996.

Goldfarb, Roz: *Careers by Design*, New York, Allworth Press, 2001.

Gordon, Sandra R.: *Great Jobs for Film Majors*, Chicago, VGM Career Books, 2004.

Graham, Duane: *The Remarkable Story of Otto Graham*, Wayne, Immortal Investments Publishing, 2004.

Green, E. and Adam, A. Virtual Gender: *Technology, Consumption, and Identity*, New York, Routledge, 2001.

Greenman, Robert: *The Adviser's Companion*, New York, Columbia Scholastic Press Association, 1991.

Griffiths, D.: *The Exclusion of Women from Technology*, London, Pluto Press, 1985.

Hall, Ken G.: *Australian Film: the Inside Story*, Sydney, Summit Books, 1980.

Hewitt, John: *Airwords: Writing for Broadcast News, Mountain View*, Oxford, Mayfield Pub. Company, 2002.

Higham, Robin: *A Guide to the Sources of United States Military History*, Hamden, Archon Books, 1975.

Hilliard, Robert L. and Michael C. Keith: *The Broadcast Century and Beyond*, Boston: Focal Press, 2001.

Hinkin, Timothy R.: *Cases in Hospitality Management: A Critical Incident Approach*, New York, Wiley, 1995.

Holloway, J. C. : *Towards a Core Curriculum for Tourism: A Discussion Paper*, London, The National Liaison Group for Higher Education in Tourism, 1995.

Horstede, G.: *Cultures and Organizations: Software of the Mind*, London, McGraw-Hill Book Company, 1991.

Hungerland, Buff: *Marketing Your Creative Portfolio*, Upper Saddle River, Prentice Hall, 2003

Jain, S. C.: *Women and Technology*, Jaipur, Rawat Publications, 1985.

Jefferson, Michael: *Breaking into Graphic Design*, New York, Allworth Press, 2005.

Jensen, Clayne R.: *Opportunities in Recreation and Leisure Careers*, Lincolnwood, VGM Career Horizons, 2000.

Jones, Sue Jenklyn: *Fashion Design*, New York, Watson-Guptill, 2002.

Kieffer, John: *The Photographer's Assistant*, New York, Allworth, 2001.

Kirkham, P.: *The Gendered Object*, Manchester, Manchester University Press, 1996.

Kissane, Sharon F.: *Career Success for People with Physical Disabilities*, Lincolnwood, VGM Career Horizons, 1997.

Kring, Robin: *Party Creations: Book of Theme Event Design*, Denver, Clear Creek Pub., 1993.

Kurzweil, R.: *The Age of Spiritual Machines*, New York, Viking, 1999.

Lavery, P.: *Tourism Marketing and Management Handbook*, New York, Prentice Hall, 1989.

Lewis, Robert C.: *Cases in Hospitality Marketing and Management*, New York, John Wiley, 1997.

MacCloskey, Monro: *How to Qualify for the Service Academies*, New York, Richards Rosen Press, 1964.

Maclay, Edgar Stanton: *A History of the United States Navy 1771-1893*, New York, Appleton Co., 1894.

Mauro, Lucia: *Careers for Fashion Plates and Other Trendsetters*, Chicago, VGM Career Horizons, 2003.

McGuire-Lytle, Erin: *Careers in Graphic Arts and Computer Graphics*, New York, Rosen, 1999.

Miller, Samuel D.: *An Aerospace Bibliography*, Washington. Office of Air Force History, 1978.

Mitchell, Leslie Scott: *Freelancing for Television and Radio*, London; Routledge, 2005.

Mogel, Leonard: *Creating Your Career in Communications and Entertainment*, Sewickley, GATF Press, 1998.

Noronha, Shonan F. R.: *Opportunities in Television and Video Careers*, Chicago: VGM Career Books, 2003.

Orlik, Peter B.: *Career Perspectives in Electronic Media*, Ames, Blackwell Pub., 2004.

Packard, Sidney: *The Fashion Business: Dynamics and Careers*, New York, Holt, Rinehart, and Winston, 1983.

Parks, Peggy J.: *The News Media*, San Diego, Lucent Books, 2002.

Paullin, C.O.: *The Navy of the American Revolution*, Cleveland, The Burrows Brothers Co., 1906.

Perna, Rita: *Fashion Forecasting*, New York, Fairchild Publications, 1987.

Rachlis, Eugene: *The Story of the U.S. Coast Guard*, New York, Random House, 1961.

Reis, Ronald A.: *Careers in Art and Graphic Design*, Hauppage, Barrons, 2001.

Rocha, Tony L.: *Careers in Magazine Publishing*, New York, Rosen, 2001.

Rubinstein, Donna: *The Modeling Life*, New York, Berkeley Publishing Group, 1998.

Satterthwaite, Frank: *The Career Portfolio Workbook*, New York, McGraw-Hill, 2003.

Seguin, James: *Media Career Guide*, Boston, St. Martin's, 2006.

Sones, Melissa: *Getting into Fashion: A Career Guide*, New York, Ballantine, 1984.

Vogt, Peter: *Career Opportunities in the Fashion Industry*, New York, Facts on File, 2002.

Wilson, Wayne: *Careers in Publishing and Communications*, Bear, Mitchell Lane, 2002.

Yager, Fred, & Jan Yager: *Career Opportunities in the Film Industry*, New York, Ferguson, 2003.

Zahler, Karen Gantz.: *Superchefs: Signature Recipes From America's New Royalty*, New York, John Wiley & Sons, 1996.

Index

D

E

F

G

H

I

J

L

M

N

O

S

T

❑❑❑